# DREAMS

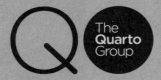

Inspiring | Educating | Creating | Entertaining

Brimming with creative inspiration, how-to projects, and useful information to enrich your everyday life, quarto.com is a favorite destination for those pursuing their interests and passions.

Copyright © 2022 by Zambezi Publishing Ltd.
Text © 2022 by Zambezi Publishing Ltd.
Unless otherwise noted on page 143, illustrations © 2022 Quarto Publishing Group USA Inc.

First published in 2022 by Wellfleet Press,
an imprint of The Quarto Group,
142 West 36th Street, 4th Floor,
New York, NY 10018, USA
T (212) 779-4972 F (212) 779-6058
**www.Quarto.com**

Wellfleet titles are also available at discount for retail, wholesale, promotional, and bulk purchase. For details, contact the Special Sales Manager by email at specialsales@quarto.com or by mail at The Quarto Group, Attn: Special Sales Manager, 100 Cummings Center Suite, 265D, Beverly, MA 01915 USA.

10 9 8 7 6 5 4 3 2 1

Library of Congress Control Number: 2021947784

ISBN: 978-1-57715-263-7

Publisher: Rage Kindelsperger
Creative Director: Laura Drew
Managing Editor: Cara Donaldson
Cover and Interior Design: Ashley Prine/Tandem Books
Editor: Elizabeth You

Printed in China

{ IN FOCUS }

# DREAMS

## ❧ Your Personal Guide ❧

### Angela Mogridge

WELLFLEET
PRESS

# CONTENTS

# INTRODUCTION

O ne minute, you are flying high above your house; the next, you are having an in-depth conversation with a long-dead relative before you have to save everyone as your home catches fire—all of which happens during a typical night in the dream world!

We all dream, almost certainly every night; some dreams we remember vividly, and others we never recall. Some dreams will stay with us for a considerable period of time, and they can make us feel uncomfortable and vulnerable. Others make us happy or motivated or determined to change something. Many leave us confused as to their meaning, making little logical sense to our conscious minds.

For something that we do every night and that can have such an impact on our emotions and our mental well-being, we know very little definitively about dreams. What is known for sure is that many people are fascinated by the subject and have lots of questions about dreams and dreaming.

For centuries people have puzzled over the meaning of dreams. The earliest civilizations thought that dreams were a link between our world and that of the gods, while the Greeks and Romans believed that dreams had prophetic powers and predicted the future. By the nineteenth century, the fields of psychology and science had started to investigate the phenomenon.

This book will look at some of those questions and attempt to find answers from various sources. There is a comprehensive dream directory so that you can find out the meanings of some of your strangest dreams.

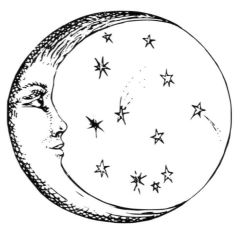

By the end of your journey, you will have a greater understanding of dreaming, including both the science behind it and the mysticism attached to it.

# Some Common Questions about Dreams

Let's start with some of the basic questions everyone has about dreams, and the short answers to them.

## Why do we dream?

This is perhaps the most challenging question to answer! Neuroscientists, psychologists, spirit guides, and mystics all have their explanations and theories for why we dream—many of which we will look at during our journey through this book.

## What is a dream?

A dream can be described as a series of dramatized images and visions that occur in our minds during certain stages of sleep—specifically during the *rapid eye movement* stage of dreaming, known as REM. During our journey through this exploration of dreams, we will learn about the stages that our minds and bodies go through during sleep and what happens to our brains when we dream.

## Why can't I always remember my dreams?

Sometimes you *can* remember your dreams, but sometimes you remember only fragments, and it might be hours after waking that you find parts of a dream coming back to you. There are even times when we can't be sure whether a memory is just that—a real memory or a dream. However, scientists believe that you are more likely to remember your dream if you wake up during the REM dreaming stage.

## How long do dreams last?

A dream can last for a few seconds or as long as thirty minutes. Sleep scientists believe that the average person has three to five dreams per night, with some people experiencing up to seven in a night. Over a lifetime, a person might dream for up to six whole years!

## Are there different types of dreams?

There are probably as many different types of dreams as there are dreamers! We all likely experience a range of different dreams during our lifetime. There are fantastical dreams, which seem to have no bearing on real life; logical, practical dreams, which are exactly like real life; dreams that make us feel happy, sad, scared, or unsettled, and so many more.

## What are nightmares?

Nightmares are dreams that create feelings of fear and panic—often resulting in us waking suddenly, sometimes with a scream! Nightmares may be caused by stress, anxiety, or post-traumatic stress disorder (PTSD), but they are just as likely to have no obvious source or cause.

Children tend to have more nightmares than adults, but everyone will experience a "bad dream" at some point in their lives. Horrible nightmares are often referred to as *night terrors*—and can lead to conditions such as sleepwalking, insomnia (the inability to begin to or continue to sleep), or sleep paralysis—the feeling of being awake but unable to move.

## What are lucid dreams?

Lucid dreams can occur during the late stages of REM sleep when you are aware you are asleep but can, to some extent, control events that happen in your dream. Some people dedicate time to learning how to lucid dream, believing that, among other things, lucid dreaming increases confidence and creativity.

## Do dreams have meaning?

This is almost as tricky a question to answer as "how and why do we dream?" and there are nearly as many theories and opinions about the meaning or otherwise of dreams. Check out chapter six in this book to see what the most common dreams might mean.

## Do animals dream?

Because all mammals experience REM while sleeping, all can dream. In their 7–9 hours of sleep each night, humans experience about 2 hours of REM. Comparatively, cats sleep an average of 13 hours a day, getting as much as 8 hours of REM. Research has found that African elephants sleep only 2 hours a day, so they 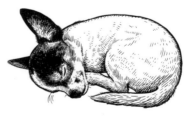 sometimes don't reach REM at all. And some animals, such as dolphins, only sleep with half of their brain at a time, so they can continue swimming while they sleep.

## DREAM VISION

Blind people who lose sight before the age of seven are likely to dream in senses other than sight.

Not all sighted people dream in color—some always dream in black and white.

## What about babies?

It might come as no surprise that, because babies spend more than half their time sleeping, they are likely to be big dreamers. Since they can't tell what they've dreamed, it's hard for researchers to know. Studies suggest that children begin to dream similarly to adults between the age of three and seven. The elderly, on the other hand, are thought to spend less than a fifth of their time asleep—with an associated drop in the rate of dreaming.

Those are the basics on dreaming. As you read this book, you will find much more information on many of these topics..

## Enclosed Dream Wall Chart

Included in this book is a wall chart that serves as a quick and handy reference guide containing an abridged list of some of the most common symbols that appear in dreams.

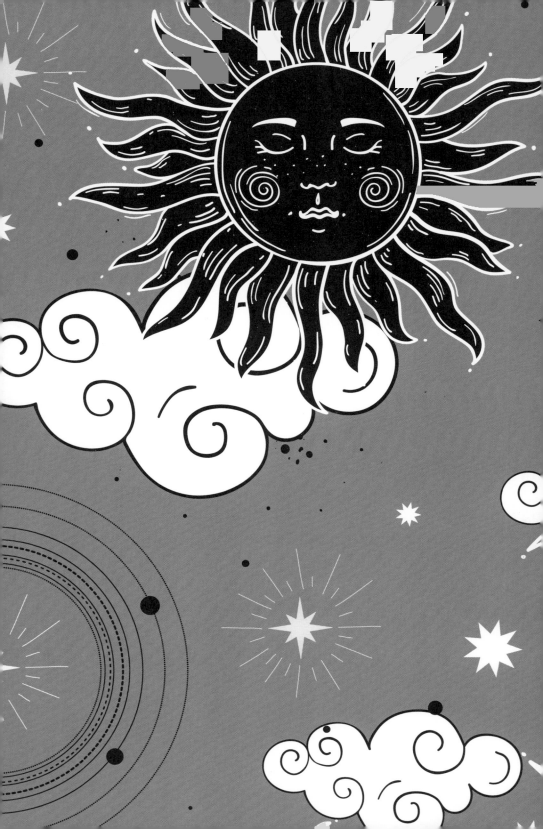

## PART I
# DREAM THEORY

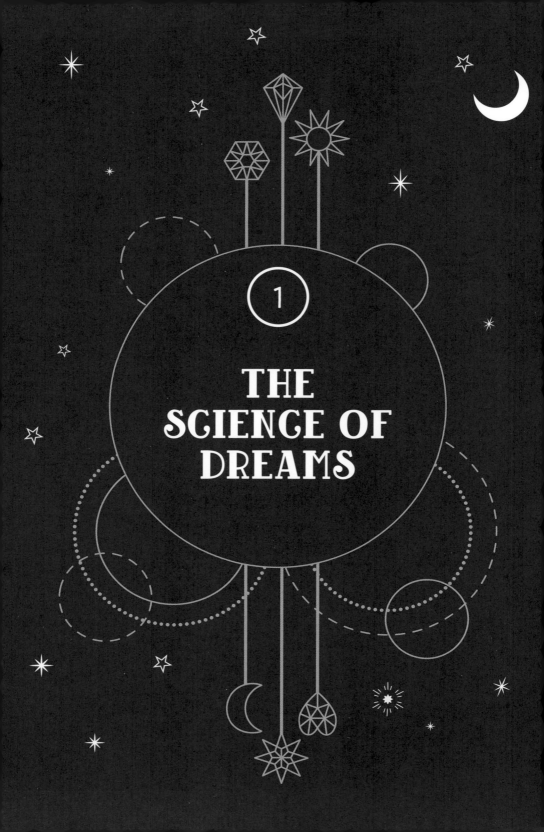

# 1

# THE SCIENCE OF DREAMS

To understand how we dream and the science of dreaming, it is necessary briefly to introduce our brains!

The brain is one of the largest and most complicated organs in the human body. It comprises many different areas, each of which performs a specialist task, but, importantly, work together:

- The **cortex** is the outermost layer of brain cells and controls thinking and voluntary movements.
- The **brain stem,** between the spinal cord and the rest of the brain, controls breathing and sleep.
- The **basal ganglia** are a cluster of structures in the brain's center that coordinate messages to the brain.
- The **cerebellum,** at the base and back of the brain, is responsible for coordination and balance.
- The **limbic system** consists of the **amygdala** and the **hippocampus,** situated at the top of the brain stem. The parts of the limbic system are responsible for emotions and motivation.
- The brain is also divided into several lobes:
    - The **frontal lobes** are responsible for problem solving, judgment, and motor function.
    - The **parietal lobes** control sensation, handwriting, and body position.
    - The **temporal lobes** are responsible for memory and hearing.
    - The **occipital lobes** contain the visual processing system of the brain.

# The Biology of Dreams

By the end of your journey with this dream guide, you will realize that there is very little agreement about dreams, such as their meaning, their function, and their benefits or otherwise. However, with a greater scientific understanding of sleep has come a general agreement on *how* we dream.

While sleeping, our bodies and minds go through five different stages:

As we fall asleep at stage one, our muscle movement slows down, and as our breathing and heart rate slow, we move into stage two. Stage one and two of our sleep cycle last a total of about thirty minutes, and during these stages, it is

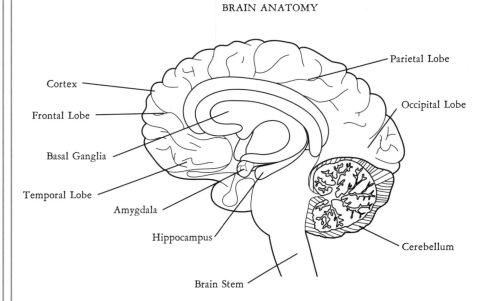

BRAIN ANATOMY

Cortex

Frontal Lobe

Basal Ganglia

Temporal Lobe

Amygdala

Hippocampus

Brain Stem

Parietal Lobe

Occipital Lobe

Cerebellum

easy for us to be roused. Muscles and brain waves continue to slow as we move further and further into a deep sleep. However, by stage five, our heart rate increases, and our brain waves speed up, and behind our closed eyelids, our eyes flutter rapidly—hence this stage is known as *rapid eye movement*, or *REM*.

It is at this stage—approximately eighty minutes after falling asleep—that we start to dream. We spend around 15 to 35 percent of our sleep in stage five, meaning that we have about four or five periods of REM each night. The first REM period of the night is likely to last around ten minutes, with each subsequent REM session lasting longer and longer—the final once lasting up to an hour. Dreams can occur during the other stages of sleep, but they will be less vivid and less memorable.

## Brain Waves

Brain waves are the flow and changes in the electrical currents in our brain. We often talk of having a brain wave, when in fact there are five brain waves—gamma, beta, alpha, theta, and delta (these are in order of highest frequency to lowest). Each of these waves has a specific purpose and causes us to behave and think in different ways. These brain waves do not stop just because we are sleeping—in fact, they are working as hard as when we are awake. Our brain's ability to be flexible and transition through each brain wave state smoothly affects how we deal with stress, focus, and even sleep. Our brains move from one type of brain wave to another and back again throughout the day, and one will be more dominant than the others, depending on our state of consciousness.

## Gamma Waves
- Important for learning, memory, and information processing.
- People who have learning difficulties tend to have lower gamma activity than others.
- You can increase your gamma waves through meditation.
- Too much gamma activity can lead to anxiety and stress.
- Too little can lead to depression and learning and memory problems.

## Beta Waves
- These are important for conscious thought and logical thinking.
- Coffee, energy drinks, and stimulants increase beta waves.
- Too much beta activity can lead to high arousal, anxiety, stress, high adrenaline, and inability to relax.
- Too little beta activity might cause depression, daydreaming, or poor cognition.

## Alpha Waves
- Alpha waves help us calm down and relax.
- They are the bridge between conscious awareness and subconscious sleep.
- If we become very stressed, we can experience "alpha blocking," during which there is excessive beta wave activity and not enough alpha wave activity.
- Too much alpha activity can cause daydreaming, lethargy, and being too relaxed.
- Too little may lead to anxiety, insomnia, and stress.
- Some antidepressants, alcohol, and marijuana increase alpha waves.

## Theta Waves
- Theta waves are connected to daydreaming and restorative sleep, emotions, and deep feelings.
- A healthy amount of theta activity improves a person's intuition and

creativity and can put a person into a deeply relaxed, semi-hypnotic state at times.
- Too much theta activity can result in hyperactivity, impulsiveness, and inattentiveness.
- Too little theta wave activity may lead to stress, anxiety, and emotional distress.

## Delta Waves

- These are the slowest of the five brain waves and are more active in children and babies.
- As we get older, we tend to produce fewer and fewer delta waves.
- These waves are associated with deep relaxation and restorative, healing sleep. They also help to regulate heartbeat and digestion while we are asleep.
- Delta waves are responsible for that lovely feeling we sometimes get when we feel fully refreshed after a good sleep.
- A brain injury can result in too much delta wave activity. Excessive delta action can also lead to learning difficulties and lack of focus.
- Too little delta wave activity may cause poor sleep, poor immunity, feeling run-down.
- Sleep can increase delta waves.

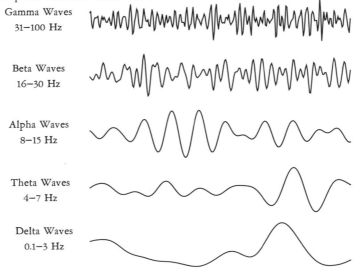

Gamma Waves
31–100 Hz

Beta Waves
16–30 Hz

Alpha Waves
8–15 Hz

Theta Waves
4–7 Hz

Delta Waves
0.1–3 Hz

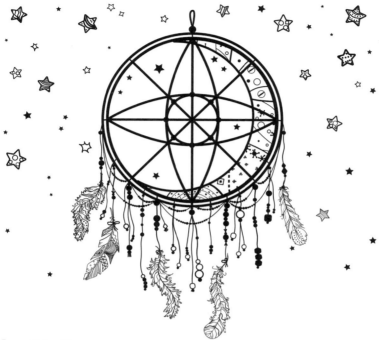

# Why We Dream

While science has yet to offer a definitive answer as to why we dream, there are certainly a number of intriguing theories out there.

## The Threat-Simulation Theory

One theory sees dreaming as an ancient biological defense mechanism within the brain that has enabled human beings to survive and evolve. Some scientists argue that our brains repeatedly simulate threats and dangers to our safety and survival when we are asleep. This repetition increases the neuro-cognitive abilities that enable us to perceive and avoid threats and dangers. So, in essence, scary dreams or ones involving danger help keep us alert to the dangers around us and enable us to seek safety when threatened.

The more that actual threatening events are experienced by an individual while awake, the greater their threat-simulation response and the greater likelihood of them having aggressive, frightening, and threatening dreams. This seems to be confirmed by research carried out by a Finnish research team led by Katja Valli. The team analyzed the dream content of severely traumatized Kurdish refugee children and non-traumatized Finnish children. The severely

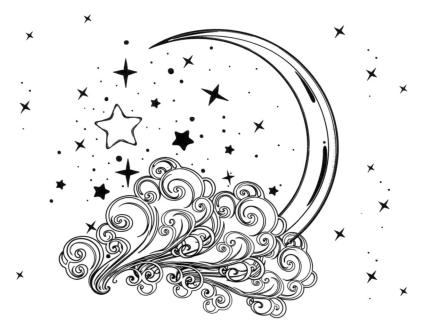

traumatized children reported a much greater incidence of severe, threatening dreams than what was experienced by the non-traumatized children.

## Activation-Synthesis Hypothesis

Harvard scientists Allan Hobson and Robert McCarley published their activation-synthesis hypothesis in 1977. Their theory states that dreams don't actually mean anything; they are merely electrical brain impulses that pull random images, memories, and thoughts together while we are asleep. A dream is our brain's attempt to make sense of all this subconscious activity. Our brains are active even when we are asleep (see the section above on brain waves). The pulling together of the imagery and thoughts is part of how our brains take the opportunity to have a "cleanup" during sleep—to organize and file away all the neural activity stimulated during the day.

When we sleep, especially when we reach the REM stage, specific brain circuits are activated, causing the limbic system to become more active. The parts of the limbic system related to emotions, feelings, and memories are especially stimulated. The activation-synthesis hypothesis speculates that the brain is programmed to give meaning to things, so it attempts to find meanings for the feelings, emotions, and memories activated, resulting in dreaming.

After experiencing a dream and waking up, individuals then construct "dream stories" or interpretations of their dreams to make sense of and give meaning to them.

According to Hobson, there are five characteristics that most dreams share:

1. **Intense emotions.** Our dreams can sometimes stir up intense emotions, in particular anxiety, fear, or even surprise. These can interrupt our dream and sleep and wake us abruptly.

2. **Disorganization and illogic.** Many of our dreams are simply bizarre—having no beginning or ending, being inconsistent over time and place, and involving groups of people who don't know one another in the real world.

3. **The acceptance of strange dream content.** Indeed, while dreaming, we tend to accept what is happening and do not question the logic of the dream. Thus, even on waking, while we may be confused and even curious for a little while (if we remember the dream), we are likely to move on quite quickly without further investigating the dream content.

4. **Strange sensations.** Dreamers often experience strange sensations, from the ability to fly, to the sense of falling off a cliff, to the inability to move, and we often feel sensations within our dreams that we don't experience in our conscious life.

5. **Difficult to remember.** The memory of a dream decreases rapidly on waking up. As many as 95 percent of dreams are forgotten on awaking.

> The brain is so inexorably bent upon the quest for meaning that it attributes and even creates meaning when there is little or none in the data it is asked to process.
>
> —Allan Hobson

## Information Processing Theory

George Miller developed the information processing theory in the 1950s. The idea compares the human brain with a computer and states that the information we give to the brain (emotions, imagery, feelings, experiences) is then filtered into our short-term and long-term memories. According to Miller, these memories are organized and filed in our brains while we are asleep, so this is what dreaming is: how our brains organize our memories.

This theory has also become known as self-organization theory, as it ranks our memories according to importance or value. Thus, when we dream, helpful, good, important, or valuable memories are made more robust, while the less valuable ones fade away.

Miller's work has led to further research, including studies that have found that we improve our skills concerning complex tasks the more we dream about those tasks. So, for example, we can become better drivers if learning to drive features heavily in our dreams. This makes sense, given that other studies have found that during REM sleep (the stage of sleep in which dreams occur), low-frequency theta waves are dominant—as they are when we are learning and remembering information when we are awake. However, this view is not shared by all neurobiologists.

## Reverse Learning

In 1983, Francis Crick and Graeme Mitchison proposed that the brain's memory system is easily overloaded (think about the number of different things you do every day and the amount of additional information you have to process each day). As a result, our brains fill up with "cognitive debris," as they called

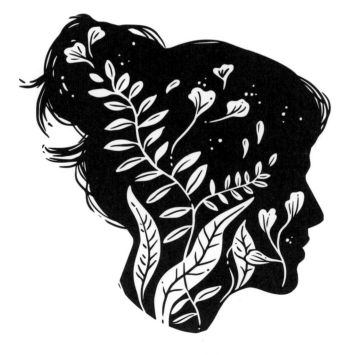

it—multiple excess items of data that clog up the brain's systems. To eliminate this cognitive debris, humans experience "dream-laden" REM sleep. Therefore, Crick and Mitchison's conclusion was that dreams have no meaning other than helping clear the brain of unnecessary memories. As Crick and Mitchison stated, "We dream to forget," a form of reverse learning, whereby we unlearn the experiences that we do not need to remember.

## Emotional Regulation Dream Theory

This theory claims that we dream to help us deal with our emotions in a safe space, which is when we sleep. During particularly vivid dreaming, the amygdala and the hippocampus within our brains are very active. These are the two areas of the brain most closely associated with processing information and moving it from short-term to long-term memory. Therefore, the thought is that we use our dream time to sort through our emotions and memories—retiring those that are not useful right now into our long-term memory. Similar research has confirmed this hypothesis, finding a link between our ability to control and process our emotions and the amount of REM sleep we get. So it would seem that the deeper we sleep and the more times we go into the REM stage, and thus the more we dream, the better we are at keeping our emotions in check.

One final biological theory to consider is that dreams are a response to external stimuli. For example, real-world noise such as a dog barking or a baby's cry while we are asleep won't always wake us. However, sometimes the external noise results in our brains trying to interpret and understand the noise, and this creates dreams in which these noises or the sources of these noises exist.

✳ ✳ ✳

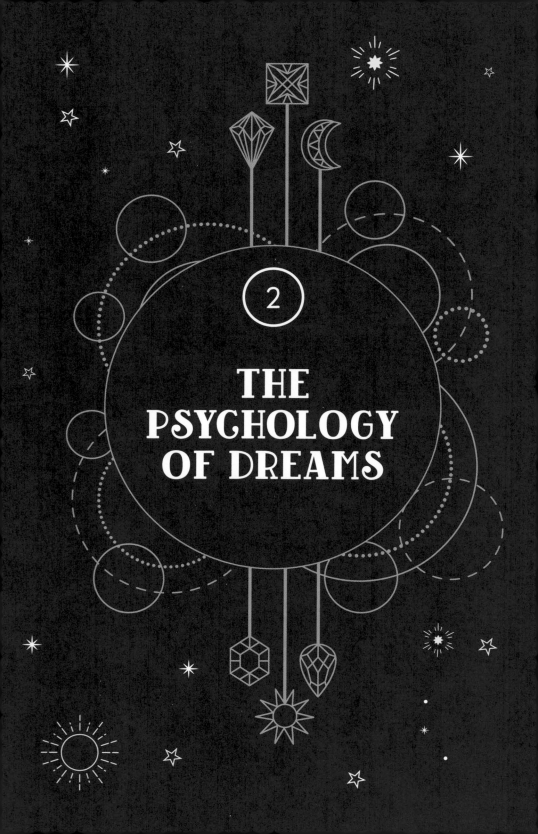

# 2

# THE PSYCHOLOGY OF DREAMS

Dreams and their causes, functions, and meanings have been a popular focus of psychologists for hundreds of years. All of the major schools of psychological thought and some very well-known psychologists have different ways of explaining dreams and their origin.

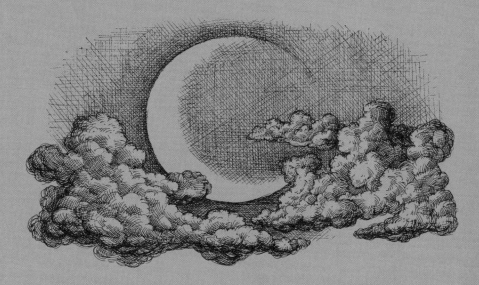

## The Psychodynamic Approach

The psychodynamic approach is a psychological theory associated with Sigmund Freud (1856–1939) and his followers. It explains human behavior as based upon the interaction of conscious and unconscious drives and forces within an individual. A basic tenet of the psychodynamic approach is that our behavior, emotions, and feelings are affected by unconscious motives and our past experiences, the memories of which are stored in our unconscious minds.

Freud was a psychoanalyst, and his theories are based on the experiences of the patients who came to him for therapy for depression and anxiety disorders. Among other things that the psychodynamic approach has theories on, dreams were of particular interest to Freud. In his famous book *The Interpretation of Dreams* (1899), he claimed that dreams were symbolic "eruptions" from our deep unconsciousness. He believed that our true desires are hidden in our unconsciousness and that these repressed desires find expression in our dreams.

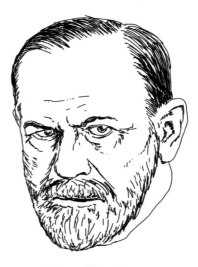

Freud believed that there were two interpretations available for each dream that we have, which are the "manifest content" (the content that we remember on waking) and

Sigmund Freud

the "latent content" (the real, underlying meaning of the dream). He claimed that a dream analyst or interpreter could differentiate between the two—thus, seeking interpretation of a dream is a worthwhile thing to do. In addition, he claimed that every dream has a connection, however minor, with something that the dreamer has experienced. Finally, he considered that dreams were made of "picture puzzles" that, through interpretation, could form a "poetic phase of the greatest beauty and significance."

Most people have multiple dreams in a night, and Freud claimed that there is a connection in the content of all dreams that happen during the same sleep. Each dream is a part of the same whole—each connected to the same unconscious desires and experiences. Interestingly, he believed that the first dream of the night was likely to be the most distorted (and perhaps less memorable) and that each subsequent dream became more distinct and more apparent as the night went on.

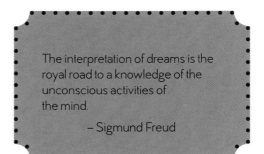

The interpretation of dreams is the royal road to a knowledge of the unconscious activities of the mind.

– Sigmund Freud

# The Cognitive Approach

Cognitive psychology looks at the way we think and understand things. For example, Calvin Hall (1909–1985) collated more than 50,000 records of dreams over several years and from around the world. From his research, he surmised that dreams represent how we see ourselves, what we think about other people, and how we view the world. In his famous work, *The Meaning of Dreams* (1966), he claimed that "the images of a dream are the concrete embodiments of the dreamer's thoughts; these images give visual expression to that which is invisible, namely conceptions."

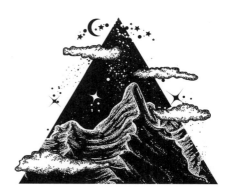

Hall identified five cognitive structures and attitudes that dreams can reveal:

1. **Conceptions of self**—How we see ourselves, the roles we play in life.
2. **Conceptions of others**—The people in our lives, how we react to their needs.
3. **Conceptions of the world**—Our environment, where we live, how we live.
4. **Conceptions of penalties**—What is allowed? What is acceptable? What is forbidden?
5. **Conceptions of conflict**—Our inner discord and how we struggle to resolve it.

So, for example, you might dream about losing all your teeth. While on the one hand, this might be dismissed as a nonsense dream, using the cognitive approach we might conclude that it has to do with your conception of yourself—that you are worried about your appearance and perhaps about losing your looks.

## The Humanist Approach

The humanist approach to dreams has some similarity with that of the psychodynamic approach discussed above. Proponents of both believe that dreaming is about a person's deeper self. However, humanists see dreams as having a meaning unique to each individual, and thus we can't generalize about the meaning of dreams. They assert that, in our conscious life, we are constantly trying to improve ourselves and reach our full potential. In addition, we are often trying to make sense of a confusing world and bring order to our lives. These things transfer to our dream world, where we are frequently at risk or in peril or facing a challenge and subconsciously trying to bring order, sense, and meaning to our dreams.

## The Behavioral Approach

The behavioral approach does not rely on mental processes that cannot be observed. Therefore, behaviorists do not focus on the memories or desires represented by dreams, unlike other psychological schools of thought. Instead, a behaviorist views a dream as an individual response to environmental stimulation, such as noise, vibrations, discomfort, or even the weather.

### Carl Jung and Dreams

Carl Jung (1875–1961), a fellow psychoanalyst and one-time collaborator of Sigmund Freud, was fascinated by the study of dreams. He started believing that the mind, body, and feelings all work together in synchronicity and form what he called "the psyche." Significantly, he proposed that dreams formed part of this psyche. Jung believed that a healthy person (both physically and mentally) needed to be in balance—an imbalance would cause illnesses such as depression. Thus, the psyche was seen as a "self-regulating system" where all the elements (thoughts, feelings, the body) had a purpose.

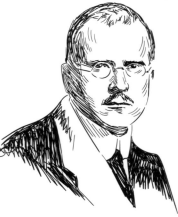

Carl Jung

Carl Jung saw dreams as the psyche's attempt at communicating something to the dreamer, and thus he placed a very high value on dreaming. He disagreed with Freud's conclusion that dreams were about hidden, repressed desires. In contrast, Jung felt that dreams expressed things quite openly. As he argued: "They do not deceive, they do not lie, they do not distort…they are invariably seeking to express something that the ego does not know and does not understand."

He also disagreed with Freud's view that dreams needed to be interpreted, instead suggesting that our dreams integrate our conscious and unconscious lives through what he called *individuation*—which singles them out as individual to the dreamer.

Psychologists may never agree on whether dreams serve a real purpose. However, dream interpretation provides interesting insights in our psychology.

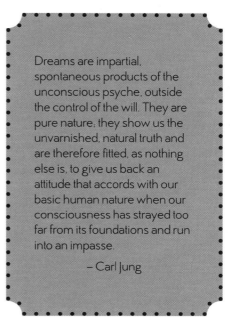

Dreams are impartial, spontaneous products of the unconscious psyche, outside the control of the will. They are pure nature, they show us the unvarnished, natural truth and are therefore fitted, as nothing else is, to give us back an attitude that accords with our basic human nature when our consciousness has strayed too far from its foundations and run into an impasse.

– Carl Jung

❋ ❋ ❋

# 3

# DREAMS AND SPIRITUALITY

Long before scientists began investigating dreams, various religions were exploring dreams in their own way. From initiation rituals to relating dreams to beliefs, faith, morality, and fate, most religions have made use of the dream world to explain what is sometimes inexplicable.

## In Islam

Islam explains that when we sleep, our souls partially or temporarily leave our bodies. The act of sleeping is a small death, where the body is present and the soul is elsewhere.

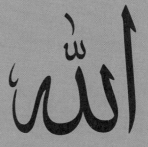

Islam categorizes dreams into three types:
1. A vision, or true dream that is from God.
2. A false dream from the devil.
3. A meaningless, standard dream from our subconscious thoughts.

### A Vision

True dreams are given either to those who are righteous or to those who will benefit spiritually from a message delivered by a vision.

### A False Dream

This is usually a nightmare sent by the devil and should not be shared with anyone. Followers were told that in the event of such a dream, they should seek refuge with God and dry spit three times to their left and three times to their right.

### A Meaningless Dream

This is differentiated from the vision and from the false dream by the way it makes the recipient feel. A vision makes the dreamer feel a sense of inspiration from God, while a false dream creates a scared and anxious feeling. A meaningless dream, on the other hand, carries no significant feeling and will likely not be remembered.

## Déjà Vu

Have you ever had the impression that you have lived through the present situation before, been somewhere that you know you have never visited and yet felt it was familiar, or that you have experienced something before that gives you a strange feeling of familiarity? Islam has explored the subject of déjà vu in some detail. It teaches that time is a creation of God, and so in God's view, the future has already happened. God is capable of transporting someone into the future and then back to the present again. The person lives normally until that point in time when they experience the déjà vu feeling of being in this place or time once again.

# In Christianity

One Christian view is that the purpose of dreams is to draw us closer to God because dreams show us how to avoid the things that come between us and God. Dreams can also reveal what we need or where we should try to go in life. God wants us to be happy and to have trust and faith in him, so if someone has a disturbing dream, they should pray to God and ask for clarification and they will receive an answer, although it may take a while before the answer comes through or becomes clear.

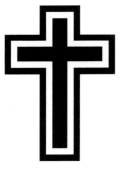

The first book of the New Testament recalls four dreams that Joseph received relating to the birth and early life of Jesus. First, Joseph is told that Mary's child was conceived by the Holy Spirit and that he should not be afraid of marrying her. In the second dream, Joseph is warned to leave Bethlehem and flee to Egypt. The third dream tells him that it is safe to return to Israel, and the final dream tells him to go to Galilee rather than Judea.

Justin Martyr, one of the earliest Christian philosophers, believed that dreams were sent by spirits. This gave weight to his argument that the human soul lives on after the death of the body. To him dreams gave us "direct spiritual communication with nonphysical realities." Irenaeus, bishop of Lyon, agreed with Justin Martyr and used this view to add weight to his argument that reincarnation did not exist. In his view, if reincarnation were real, we would remember our dreams from our previous existences.

As Christianity developed over the centuries, Christians saw dreams in different lights. Thomas Aquinas, the medieval theologian, was not originally a believer in the importance of dreams. He argued that the only sources of human knowledge were experience and rational thought—not a message or vision in a dream. However, near the end of his life, as he was finishing his great work, *Summa Theologica*, he experienced a vision in a dream that he took to be direct divine communication. This shook him to his core and led him to claim, "I can do no more. Such things have been revealed to me that all I had written seemed like straw, and I now await the end of my life."

The Reformation saw the splitting of Western Christianity into Protestantism and the Roman Catholic Church. It also saw a moving away from an acceptance of dreams and visions to a more rational approach to church doctrine. This has, in the main, remained the central view of the church, whether Protestant or Catholic, ever since. However, there are still people within the religion who believe that God speaks to them through their dreams.

## The Revelation That Led to "Amazing Grace"

In the eighteenth century, John Newton was a respected member of the Christian church in England, but before he found the church, he had been a slave trader. In the early days of his slave trade career, Newton had a dream in which he was aboard a ship in Venice harbor. A person approached him and gave him a ring, warning him to keep the ring safe in order to stay healthy and happy. In the dream a second person arrived, who persuaded him to drop the ring in the water, having convinced him that it was stupid to depend on a ring for his happiness. As soon as the ring hit the water, a fire burst in the mountains above Venice. The second person had been the tempter who made him throw away God's mercy, and as a consequence all he had facing him was the fires of hell. The first person, however, went into the water to retrieve the ring. The fire immediately stopped, and the person stated that Newton could not be trusted to keep the ring himself, but it would be kept safe for him for when he needed it. Newton soon forgot all about the dream, until, years later he found himself in a dangerous position where he "stood helpless and hopeless upon the brink of an awful eternity." He remembered his dream, called on the power of the Lord, and survived. He later wrote the words to the famous hymn "Amazing Grace," referring to the grace of God that he himself had experienced.

# In Hinduism

In Sanskrit, the language of Hinduism, the dream state is known as *Swapna* and is one of the four states of being:

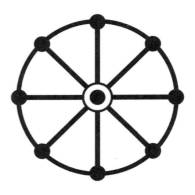

1. **Jagrit**—waking.
2. **Supta**—dreamless sleep.
3. **Swapna**—dream state.
4. **Turiya**—transcendent state.

According to Hinduism, there are seven different types of dream:

1. **Drsta**—seen. A dream that resembles or recalls things we have seen during our waking state.
2. **Sruta**—heard. A dream in which we can hear sound.
3. **Anubhuta**—experienced. Dreams in which we are aware of our five senses.
4. **Prarthita**—inner desires and wants. When we dream about something that we have desired or longed for in our waking state.
5. **Kalpita**—imagination. When our dream is full of fantasy and imaginative symbols.
6. **Bhavita**—manifested. A dream about something that has actually happened.
7. **Dosaja**—temperamental. A dream caused by an imbalance in the temperaments or emotions.

Dreams can be further categorized as *aphala* (which have no impact on the dreamer's life) or *phala* (where they do have an impact or an influence); and *subha* (a pleasant dream) or *asubha* (an unpleasant dream).

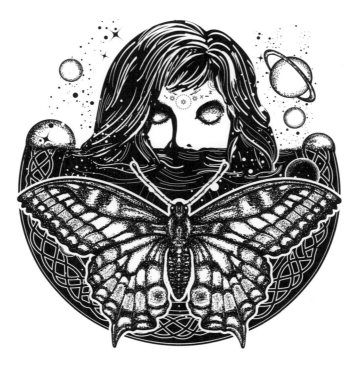

# In Judaism

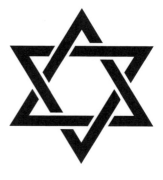

In Jewish thought, dreams are significant and can also be out-of-body experiences relaying important messages to the receiver. The Talmud, the central text of Judaism, states that "the realization of all dreams follows the mouth." Thus, the importance of the dream depends on the individual interpretation of the dream. There is no such thing as a positive or negative dream because a dream is simply *interpreted* as positive or negative. The Talmud does, however, also claim that dreams are "one-sixtieth prophetic." It could be said, therefore, that in Judaism there is a difference between "ordinary" dreams and prophetic dreams. The former is open to interpretation by the dreamer, while the latter gives the dreamer insight into the future. The Talmud also says that a dream that is not interpreted is the same as an unopened letter; therefore Jacob, and other receivers of dreams, should seek the meanings of their dreams.

# In Buddhism

A central story in Buddhism revolves around a dream. Queen Maya, the mother of Buddha, dreamed that a six-tusked elephant pierced her side with one of his tusks. This then produced an immaculate conception. The queen interpreted this dream to mean that the resulting child (Buddha) would become a monarch with domain across the world.

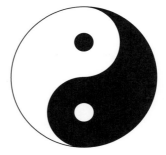

According to the Buddhist sage Nagasena, there are three organic causes of dreams:

1. Wind.
2. Bile.
3. Phlegm.

In Buddhism, dreams are creations of the mind. Every single thought we ever have is stored in our subconscious, and when we sleep some of these thoughts become activated and are replayed in our dreams. Other dreams can be set off by internal or external influences—for example, a heavy meal or stormy weather—and the subconscious mind reacts to these disturbances in the form of dreams. These two forms of dreams are deemed by Buddhism to be insignificant and not requiring interpretation.

What *does* require interpretation are dreams that are prophetic. These foretell an impending significant incident for the recipient. These dreams are brought to us by *devas*, who are the spirits of friends and family and others who have died and have been reborn but are invisible to us. The devas are keeping a watch over their loved ones and appear in a prophetic dream to warn them or prepare them for a coming incident. These dreams can warn us of danger or prepare us for good news. The messages or warnings that our devas give us in our dreams are symbolic and metaphoric rather than obvious—and so need to be interpreted.

Buddhists believe in *karma*—or cause and effect. An example of karma would be if you do good, good will come to you, but if you do bad, you should expect a bad experience in return. When karma is "about to ripen," and what we did in a previous life is about to have its reaction, a vivid dream might

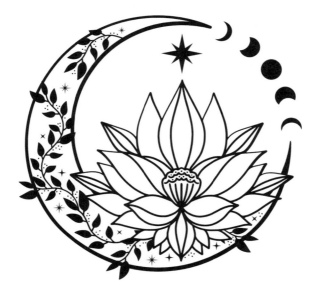

appear to a person. This dream is an expression of what is about to happen, be it bad or good. This only happens occasionally and not to everybody.

Another form of dream important to Buddhists is the one that occurs when two individuals communicate telepathically with each other. Very occasionally, when the mind is at rest or asleep, if both people concentrate hard, it is sometimes possible for them to communicate through a dream. However, it should be noted that Buddhas do not dream, and this is because they are truly enlightened and have no anxieties, negative thoughts, cravings, or unfulfilled wishes that might cause a dream to occur.

❋ ❋ ❋

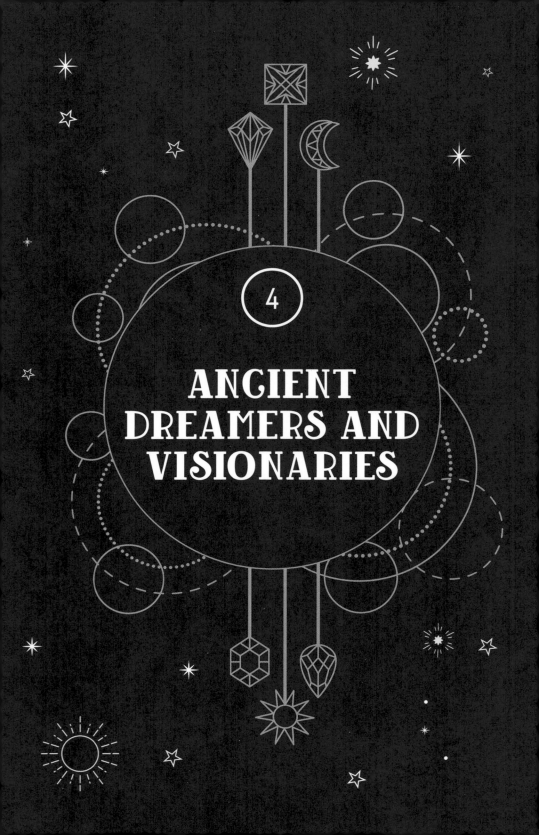

4

# ANCIENT DREAMERS AND VISIONARIES

Here are some stories and myths about sleeping, dreams, and visions from times gone by, starting with a bit more about the biblical dreams touched on in the previous chapter, and looking at ancient ideas from various places. While visions are not precisely dreams—they are experienced when a person is awake—they do have a dreamlike quality and can be described as waking dreams. The following stories show the importance (or lack of it) given to dreams and visions in ancient times.

## Biblical Dreamers

The Bible describes a number of dreamers and their dreams. The dreams were reported to have come directly from God or from a messenger of the Lord in the form of an angel. Some dream interpreters were priests, while others were people who had psychic and psychological gifts, but they all claimed that they were channeling the word of God. For instance, Isaiah and Ezekiel were both famous for their prophetic dreams, while a dream interpreter told Saul that he would become the king of Israel.

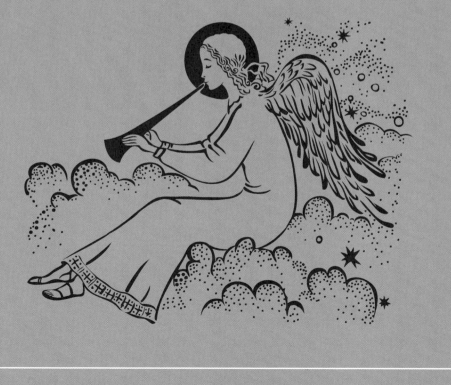

## Jacob's Ladder

In this famous story, Jacob dreamed that he saw a ladder leading up to heaven, with angels walking up and down it. He also dreamed that God told him that a year is but as a day. This may be a direct reference to an astrological technique called progressions, which are still used to this day, in which the movement of the planets during a day can be used to show the changes that take place during the course of a year.

## Joseph

Joseph of the Old Testament had a very interesting life, partly due to his knack of attracting attention and showing off in a way that irritated people. Put this alongside his ability to interpret his own prophetic dreams, and we can see how easy it was for him to land himself in hot water.

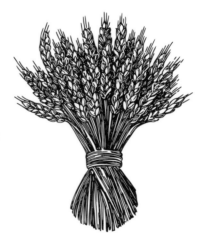

As a youngster, Joseph was helping on the family farm by tying up sheaves of wheat, and his sheaf stood up proudly while those of his brothers flopped over and appeared to bow down to his. He told his family that he interpreted this as meaning that one day his brothers would bow down to him. This didn't endear him to his brothers.

He also told his family that he had dreamed that the sun, moon, and eleven stars bowed down to him, and this was interpreted even by his indulgent father, Jacob, as yet another cheeky inference that his parents and brothers would have to bow down before him. His brothers did not appreciate Joseph or his dreams, and the outcome of this episode was that the brothers took him to Egypt and left him there, whereupon Joseph became a servant. A little later, Joseph spent some time in prison, but while there he successfully interpreted a couple of other temporary inmates' dreams. Word of this skill eventually reached the ears of the pharaoh, who was himself being troubled by a couple of very insistent dreams. Joseph interpreted the pharaoh's dreams for him, after which he became part of the pharaoh's court, eventually achieving high office.

## The Pharaoh's Dream

The Old Testament of the Bible tells of two dreams that Joseph interpreted for the pharaoh. In the first, the pharaoh dreamed that he was standing by the Nile.

> *Seven fine-looking, fat cows were coming up out of the Nile, and they grazed in the reeds. Then seven bad-looking, thin cows were coming up after them from the Nile, and they stood beside the other cows at the edge of the river. The bad-looking, thin cows ate the seven fine-looking, fat cows. Then Pharaoh woke up. Then he fell asleep again and had a second dream: There were seven heads of grain growing on one stalk, healthy and good. Then seven heads of grain, thin and burned by the east wind, were sprouting up after them. The thin heads swallowed up the seven healthy and full heads. (Genesis 41: 2-7)*

Joseph told the pharaoh that both dreams meant the same thing: there would be seven years of bumper-crop harvests, followed by seven years of famine. He suggested that the pharaoh should appoint commissioners to make the people put aside 20 percent of each harvest during the good years so that they would be able to ride out the bad ones when they occurred.

The pharaoh took Joseph's advice, and his people got through the rough times. However, the inhabitants of surrounding countries were forced to go cap in hand to Joseph to buy what they needed for survival, and among those who petitioned him were his own family. They hadn't seen their younger

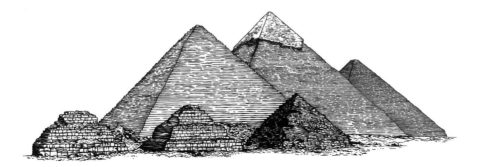

brother for many years, so while bowing down respectfully to the "Egyptian official," they didn't recognize him as *their* Joseph. Needless to say, Joseph helped them out, and after a few more adventures, he moved the whole of his family away from the poor area they had been living in to the comfort and ease of life in Egypt. It is likely that Joseph's family eventually forgave him his youthful arrogance and impertinence.

## St. Francis of Assisi

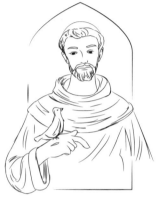

Not quite biblical but certainly Christian, Francis of Assisi was a soldier who was on his way to fight a battle when a vision turned him back. In the vision, Christ came to him and said, "Francis, Francis, go and repair my house, which as you can see is falling into ruins." St. Francis took this to mean the ruined church in which he was praying, so he stole some cloth from his father's store and sold it to pay for the repairs. When the priest refused to receive the ill-gotten gains for the repairs, Francis threw the coins away. He later embraced a life of poverty and founded several Franciscan orders, whose monks and nuns followed the gentle original teachings of Christ and turned their back on the power and pomp that the established church had become.

# Myths and Legends

Throughout history, there are many myths and legends that relate to dreams, dreamers, and the sleeping world.

## Somnus

Somnus was the god of sleep in Roman mythology. He was the twin brother of death and the son of night. He lived in a dark cave in the far west where the sun goes down—and out, to the ancient way of thinking. Lethe, the river of forgetfulness, flowed nearby and poppies and other sleep-inducing plants grew in the vicinity. Somnus is depicted as a sleeping youth holding a poppy stalk.

## Pipe Dreams

Common European poppies have been used since ancient times as a cure for sleeplessness, and they have the side effect of inducing pleasant dreams. Opium comes from large poppies, and it is well known that smoking a pipe of opium causes fantastic dreams. Hence the saying that wishful thinking that has no chance of coming into being is nothing more than "a pipe dream."

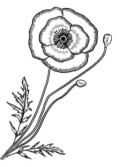

## Hermes and Morpheus

The messenger god Hermes was believed to possess magical powers over sleep and dreams, but Morpheus was considered the god of dreams, as he was the son of Hypnos, the god of sleep. Morpheus had the ability to fashion the dreams that came to sleeping people, and to enable human forms to appear in these dreams.

## Odin

According to Norse legend, Odin hung himself up in a tree by his feet for nine days and nights without eating or drinking, and as he slipped into a trance state, he noticed strange shapes forming among the roots of the tree he was hanging from. These shapes became runes, which are both an old form of alphabet and a system of divination.

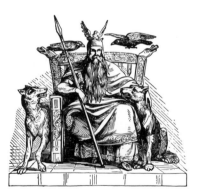

## Endymion

Endymion, the king of Elis, was absolutely gorgeous. Selene, the Greek goddess of the moon, fell in love with him. In some versions of the tale, she bore him fifty children and then put him to sleep so that she could keep him to herself. Other accounts suggest that Endymion chose to stay asleep so that he would never grow old.

## The First Dream Book

The philosopher Artemidorus, a native of Ephesus who lived in Rome from AD 138 to 180, wrote five volumes of books on the subject of dreams. Artemidorus believed that dreams were given to man to increase knowledge and for his advantage. His work has been translated into English, and much of it remains relevant.

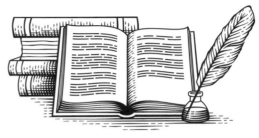

## The Oracle of Delphi

In ancient Greece, mortal oracles could communicate the word of the gods at the Temple of Apollo at Delphi. The oracles were female virgins whose job was to go into a hallucinogenic trance by either chewing "magic" leaves or throwing the leaves onto a fire and breathing in the smoke. While in this dreamy trance state, the oracles gave messages that were open to a great deal of interpretation.

## MODERN DREAM INTERPRETER: EDGAR CAYCE

Edgar Cayce's (pronounced Casey) story is a very odd one. Cayce was an unhappy young man who had to make his living selling encyclopedias. One day he lost his voice, and the medical profession couldn't help him, but a fairground hypnotist put him into a trance, during which Cayce diagnosed the cause of his ailment himself. He later learned to put himself into trances and to give correct diagnoses and holistic cures. Known as the "Sleeping Prophet," he became a renowned trance medium and allowed himself to be extensively researched.

## Nostradamus

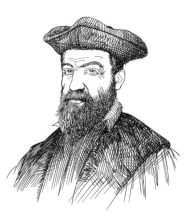

Nostradamus is well known for his collection of prophecies called *Centuries*. A student of the occult, he made his prophecies by gazing at a bowl of water and herbs and falling into a deep trance wherein he would have visions. His book is filled with mystical prophetic verses that take a great deal of interpreting, but over the centuries many believe that Nostradamus's prophecies have come true, including the Great Fire of London and the use of the atomic bomb in World War II.

## Joan of Arc

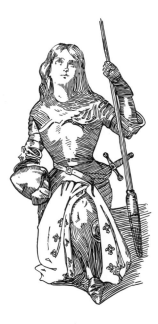

Joan of Arc (c.1412–1431), also called the Maid of Orléans, began to hear voices and see visions from the age of thirteen. She believed that St. Michael, Catherine of Alexandria, and St. Margaret were calling her to help the Dauphin and subsequent king of France, Charles. She convinced the king to allow her to lead the French troops to a decisive victory over the English during the Hundred Years' War, which ended England's claims to any part of France. Her determination carried her through some major battles, but when her siege of Paris failed in 1431, she was captured by the Burgundians, tried as a heretic, and burned at the stake. A quarter of a century later, Joan was pronounced innocent by the Catholic Church, and she was canonized in 1920 by Pope Benedict XV.

❋ ❋ ❋

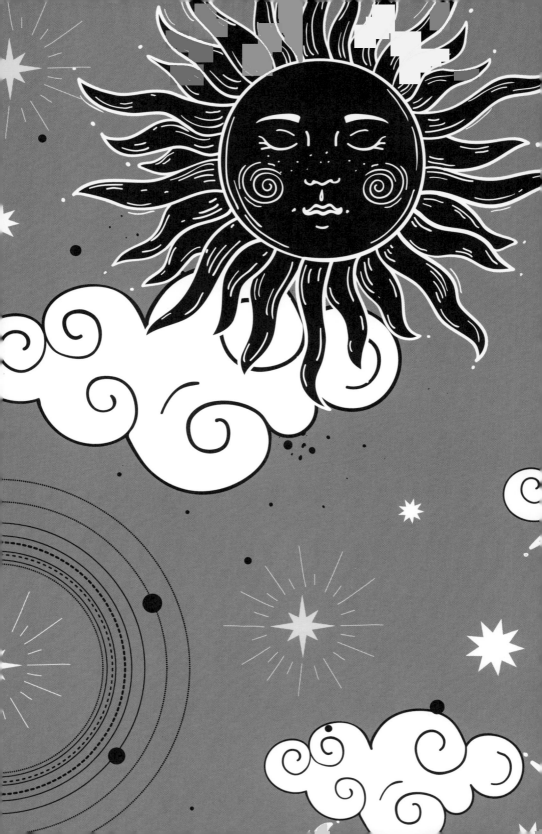

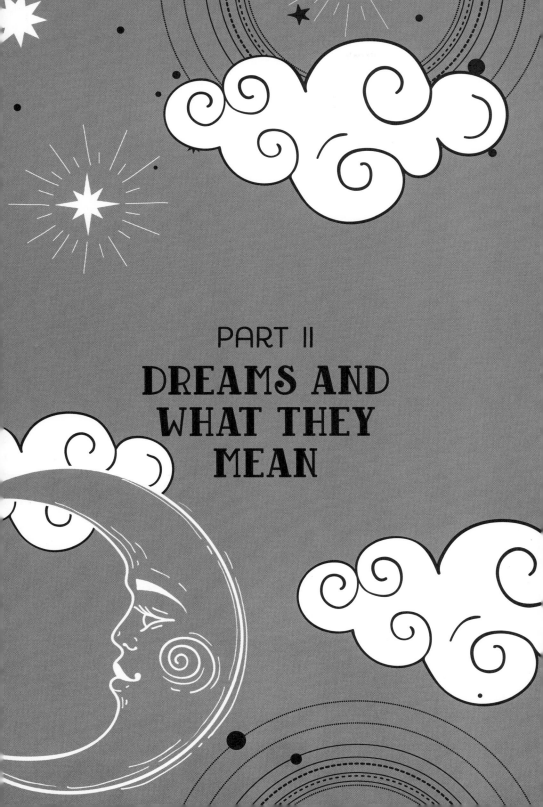

PART II

# DREAMS AND WHAT THEY MEAN

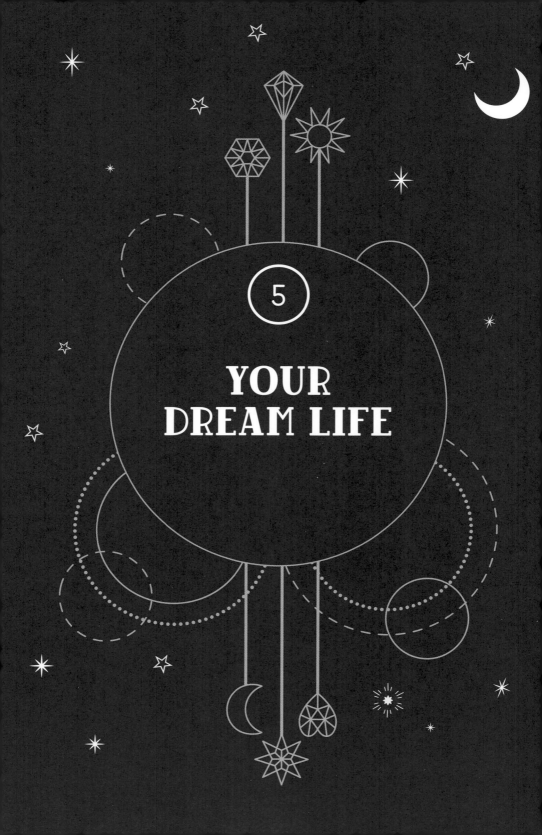

**5**

# YOUR
# DREAM LIFE

Whether you may want to remember your dreams or forget them, what follows are steps to take to do either of these things. If you want nice dreams or to experiment with the types of dreams you can induce and possibly even control, here are some scientific (and not so scientific) techniques you can try out for yourself.

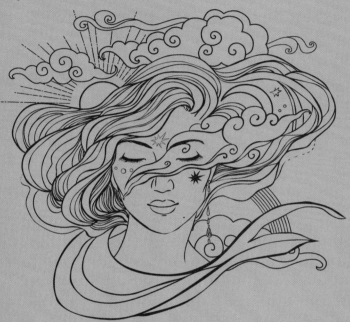

## How to Improve Your Dream Recall

It can be frustrating to wake up with a slight memory of a dream (whether it be happy, scary, or simply weird) and lose that memory almost immediately. Research indicates that we forget about 90 percent of our dreams within two minutes of waking up.

Of course, sometimes we don't want to remember a dream, but what if the dream made you feel really nice, secure, and loved? Then would you like to recall that dream?

Some people are so fascinated by their dream worlds that they go to a lot of effort every night and morning to improve their ability to recall their dreams.

Here are some ideas that you can try:

- When you go to bed, tell yourself repeatedly (try twenty or thirty times) that you will remember your dreams.
- Before you fall asleep, remind yourself of some of the dreams you have had and that you can remember. This may focus your mind on remembering, or at least paying more attention to, any dreams that you have.
- Set your alarm to go off every hour and a half. This might be better done when you don't have to get up for work in the morning! This will wake you around the times you leave REM sleep, and thus when you are likely to have dreamed.
- Keep a pen and notepad by the bed so you can write down anything you remember right away.
- Keep a sleep and dream journal to record all of your remembered dreams, and read it before sleeping each night.
- Try to wake up slowly so that you remain in a dreamlike state for as long as possible.
- Consider what type of alarm you use, because a harsh, loud one will wake you up quite dramatically, and it can put you on edge immediately. However, some great alarms are available that use bird songs or other natural sounds to wake you up and even have a sunshine type of light that will wake you up gradually.

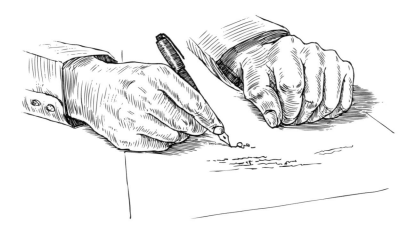

# Trauma and Stress and Dreams

Many people who have suffered from chronic stress or have experienced a traumatic event report having nightmares and vivid, recurring dreams. These dreams often add to the stress the person is suffering and make the sufferer feel that they can't switch off, even when asleep.

Of course, there are many different levels of stress and many different responses to trauma, but the most severe reaction results in a diagnosis of post-traumatic stress disorder (PTSD). PTSD is a severe anxiety disorder caused by extremely stressful, distressing, or frightening events. Examples of these events include war, serious road accidents, violent assaults, and traumatic childbirth. Among other symptoms, a person with PTSD often experiences flashbacks through nightmares and vivid dreams. Research carried out by the National Center for PTSD found that up to 96 percent of sufferers have regular nightmares, usually based around a flashback of the original trauma. These nightmares can last for months or even years after the event. Sufferers report experiencing scary dreams that make them cry out or thrash around in bed, usually culminating with waking violently in a cold sweat and with heart palpitations.

Research into PTSD has discovered that sufferers are likely to have:

- Less sleep time than non-sufferers.
- Increased instances of waking in the night.
- Decreased deep sleep.
- Increased REM sleep activity.
- Increased unsettled limb movement during sleep.

It is often necessary for a person with PTSD to seek medical and psychotherapeutic help to reduce their nightmares.

Everyday stress that is not triggered by a traumatic experience is much more common in the general population. Worries about work, financial difficulties, and relationship problems can all lead to excessive stress. After a busy, stressful day, instead of restful sleep, someone who is very stressed will often experience vivid dreams, nightmares, or disturbed sleep. This is because the mind holds on to our real-life experiences and thus can reproduce our feelings about these events during sleep. There are several ways in which we can try to reduce stress and thus reduce the probability of uncomfortable and distressing dreams:

1. **Make sure you wind down before bed.** Create a ritual for yourself—perhaps a warm bath, candles, some soft music, or an hour's reading. Be sure to turn off all electronic devices and keep off social media for at least an hour before bed.

2. **Make your bedroom a place for sleep and sex and nothing else.** If you find yourself awake into the early hours worrying, get up and take that worry somewhere else, such as to another room. Don't let your bedroom be associated with any negative feelings, stress, or anxiety.

3. **Practice relaxation techniques.** Yoga, mindfulness, meditation, and breathing exercises are excellent activities that will relax you and put you in the right frame of mind for bed.

4. **Schedule "worry" time.** Constantly telling yourself not to worry about something will have the opposite effect! Instead, allow yourself a certain amount of time, daily or weekly, to focus completely on what is worrying you—just don't do it in the bedroom. The chances are that you may actually find solutions to your worry and stress by allowing yourself this time.

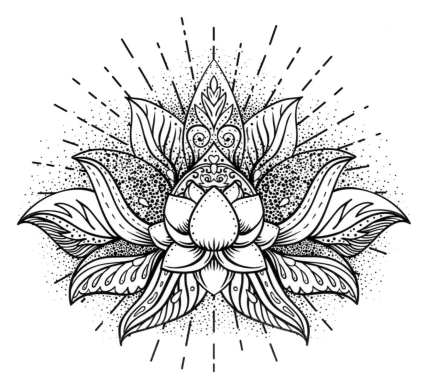

# Lucid Dreams

There are two definitions of lucid dreams. The first refers to the times when you know that you are dreaming and what's happening is not real, but it still feels real and everything is clear and lucid. (In a non-lucid dream, the sleeper is not aware that they are dreaming and events do seem super-real at the time.) The other definition of a lucid dream has to do with being able to choose what to dream about before going to sleep. Some people who have regular lucid dreams are able to exercise some degree of control over their dream—as if they were directing it.

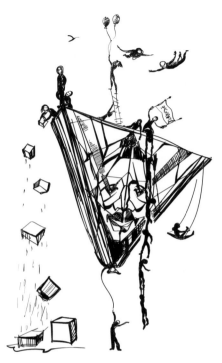

Experiencing "basic" lucid dreams where the sleeper is aware that they are dreaming is not that uncommon, and at least 23 percent of the population have one lucid dream of this kind a month. However, it is much less common to be able to control and direct a dream. As with all dreaming, lucid dreams of both types occur during periods of REM sleep—where there is very deep sleep, rapid eye movement, faster breathing, and more brain activity.

When the person knows he is dreaming, research has pinpointed action in the prefrontal cortex of the brain as being responsible. Participants in various scientific studies have displayed prefrontal cortex activity rates while they were lucid dreaming that were comparable to levels when they are awake.

As a result, some researchers refer to lucid dreamers as being in a "hybrid sleep–wake state." The prefrontal cortex of the brain is the very front of the brain and is responsible for high-level tasks such as making decisions and recalling memories. Some researchers claim that the prefrontal cortex is actually larger in those who have regular lucid dreams. This has led to suggestions that the people who are more likely to experience lucid dreams are those who are self-reflective and like to think things through.

How can scientists carry out this research on sleepers who are lucid dreaming? In most research exercises scientists use an electroencephalogram (EEG), a device to measure brain activity levels. To track eye movements (to make sure the subject has entered REM sleep), they can use an electrooculogram (EOG). Some experiments have even been carried out where the subject is asked (before sleep) to make specific eye movements while sleeping to indicate that they have a lucid dream.

## Learning to Lucid Dream

Some people believe that being able to direct a lucid dream is a skill that can be learned or nurtured, and there are a number of suggestions for developing this skill:

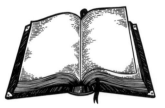

- **Dream diary.** Keeping a note of your dreams, lucid or otherwise, makes you focus daily on dreaming. Some people swear by this as a method for eventually being able to summon lucid dreams at will.
- **Reality testing.** Here you pause several times during the day to see whether you are dreaming or awake. Perhaps ask yourself if you are awake. Try to do something that would only be possible in a dream; for example, pushing your finger through your palm! The theory behind this is that doing this repeatedly over time will eventually seep into your subconsciousness. The hope is that ultimately you will be able to tell the difference between lucid and non-lucid dreams when asleep and so be able to use your powers of direction when a lucid dream does occur.
- **Wake back to bed (WBTB).** Putting an alarm on to wake you up after four or five hours, getting up, and then returning to sleep after thirty to forty minutes is said to enable some people to induce lucid dreaming. Presumably the reason for this is that the sleeper can't get a proper night's sleep, and the disturbance itself is likely to upset the equilibrium and make the sleeping person dream lucidly.
- **Mnemonic induction of lucid dreams (MILD).** With MILD you train yourself to be able to recognize the difference between dreams and reality while asleep. You need to wake up after a set period of sleep (four or five hours is optimum) and repeat the following several times:

"Next time I'm asleep, I'll remember I'm dreaming." It is thought that the constant practice of remembering to do something in the future can trigger lucid dreaming.

## The Benefits of Lucid Dreaming

Many people believe that being able to experience lucid dreams has a benefit in their conscious lives. Some of these benefits include:

- **Decreased anxiety.** It is thought that by being able to direct your lucid dream you are left with a sense of confidence and control that you can take into your conscious life. Knowing that you can shape the beginning, middle, and end of a dream may make you feel more in control of your own life and life's problems.
- **Increased creativity.** Participants in some scientific experiments with lucid dreaming abilities were able to come up with more ideas and creative solutions to problems than other participants.
- **Improved motor skills.** Research experiments have shown that it is possible to improve certain skills by practicing these skills in a lucid dream. The example used in the experiment was the tapping of fingers; lucid dreamers who practiced this in their dreams were able to tap their fingers more quickly than before.

## The Dangers of Lucid Dreaming

Lucid dreaming can, however, cause problems for some people, including:

- **Sleep disruption.** Lucid dreaming can disturb your sleep and also make you feel less rested in the morning. Also, some of the training techniques, in particular WBTB and MILD, have you deliberately waking up after four or five hours, and you might find it difficult to go back to sleep.
- **Mental health effects.** By blurring the distinction between sleep and waking, lucid dreaming may cause mental health problems for some people. Confusion, delirium, and hallucinations are examples of problems that can arise.

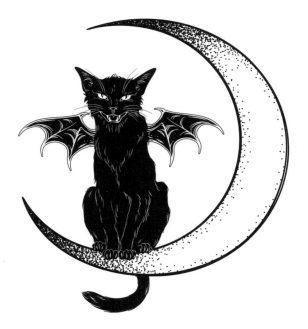

# How to Give Yourself a Nightmare!

One in every two adults experiences a nightmare at one time or another. Being pushed from a roof, chased by a wild animal, kidnapped by a monster, or watching your car running down a hill and being unable to reach it and stop it are some of the images that make us wake up in a cold sweat with a sensation of anxiety.

What factors can increase the likelihood of having a nightmare? Here is your (tongue-in-cheek) guide to how to make yourself have a nightmare:

1. **Scare yourself before bed.** We often dream of something that has been on our mind during the day, and if that happens to be a horror movie that we watched just before going to sleep, well, you can probably guess the rest!

2. **Drink alcohol.** Alcohol does initially reduce REM sleep and thus prevents you from dreaming during the first few hours of sleep, but excess alcohol can soon lead to some very weird and scary dreams later on during the night.

3. **Eat something rich, spicy, or difficult to digest.** There are various bad dream myths associated with a range of food, some of which have been debunked by scientific research. It is, however, still widely held that

rich and spicy food, which is less able to be digested by the body, if eaten close to bedtime, tends to lie in the stomach all night and then set off bad dreams. Spicy food also raises body temperature, and this can induce nightmares.

4. **Add a bit of stress to your life.** A significant amount of stress in your life, along with worry and anxiety, are perfect ingredients for bad dreams and nightmares.

5. **Take vitamin B6.** Apparently, vitamin B6 increases the level of serotonin in the bloodstream, and this can cause you to have vivid dreams that often stay in the memory for some time.

6. **Sleep on your left side or on your front.** Research carried out by the Shue Yan University in Hong Kong, China found that 41 percent of people who sleep on their left sides report experiencing bad dreams and nightmares, compared with only 15 percent of those who are right-side sleepers. And those who sleep on their fronts are more likely to dream about difficulties in breathing or of being smothered.

# Recurring Dreams

Recurring dreams are extremely common and can occur weekly, monthly, or over a period of years. It is also possible that you had the same dream numerous times before you even started recalling it.

While a recurring dream can be about anything, there are certain common themes, and researchers have found that the most common types of recurring dreams are:

- Trying to catch a flight at an airport.
- Sitting for a test or an exam at school or college.
- Dreaming about snakes.
- Being chased.
- Falling off a cliff.
- Losing all your teeth.
- Apocalyptic dreams.
- Car or airplane crashes.

You can read about some possible meanings of the symbols in your recurring dreams in the next chapter, but know that recurring dreams are often triggered by stress or exhaustion. Some people believe that their function is to deliver a message to the recipient. Keeping a dream journal, in which the first thing you do every morning is to write down what you can remember of your dream, can help in trying to work out what the dream is trying to tell you. You have to be quick, though, because we forget 90 percent of our dreams within two minutes of waking up!

## Precognitive Dreams

What if you dream of something horrible like a car crash, and it happens soon afterward? Or maybe you dream that your distant cousin turns up unannounced at a family dinner, and it happens in real life? Precognitive dreams don't have to be so precise, though, as you might awaken from a dream with a strange feeling of foreboding or fear or anxiety, and then sometime later a real-life event happens that gives you the same feelings.

It is difficult to find accurate figures for the number of people who experience precognitive dreams, and it also depends on a person's interpretation of their dream. Those who are more open to psychic experiences are more likely to interpret their dreams as precognitive, while those who are not open to such experiences are less likely to even recall such a dream.

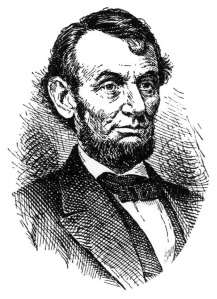

A famous example of a precognitive dream is one had by US President Abraham Lincoln in 1865. Two weeks before his death, he dreamed that there was a funeral at the White House. When, in his dream, he asked who was dead, he was told: "The president of the United States." Two weeks later he was assassinated.

# DISASTER DREAMS

◆

Precognitive dreams are rare, but they certainly do happen. For instance, there is one precognitive dream that many working psychics experienced before it happened, and that was the attack on the Twin Towers in New York City on September 11, 2001.

People who are open to having precognitive dreams usually see them as a warning. It prepares the dreamer for something that is going to happen, which, in some circumstances, allows the dreamer to make changes to prevent the event.

Not everyone believes that precognitive dreams have any psychic validity, and they look to other reasons for why such a dream can occur or be interpreted as such. So, what might cause a precognitive dream to happen? Scientific research has narrowed it down to three possible reasons:

1. **Coincidence:** Many people write off precognitive dreams to coincidence. The more dreams you have, and the more dreams you remember, the more likely it is for something to happen in real life that corresponds with something that appeared in a dream.
2. **Selective recall:** Dream research has shown that when a real-life event appears to mirror something that happened in a dream, people are more likely to remember the similarities rather than the differences.
3. **Relating the unrelated:** A good example of this would be that you have a dream that you can't necessarily recall but that has left you feeling downhearted. A couple of days later, you find out that someone you know has died, and as a result you feel sadness. Because of the similar emotions you have in real life to those that you felt in the dream, you might try to make a connection between the dream and the death.

## Night Terrors and Sleepwalking

While night terrors are not technically dreams, a small percentage of young children experience them. It can seem like they are having nightmares because they will often scream, shout, and cry while asleep. They are likely to thrash about in extreme panic and jump about, and their eyes will sometimes be open, but they are not awake. A night terror episode can last several minutes, and a child can experience more than one in the same night. They may not recognize you if you try to comfort them, and it may take some time for them to calm down. Fortunately, they usually have no memory of the night terror the next day.

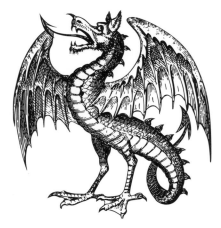

While the exact causes of night terrors are not known, it is thought that the following factors can trigger an episode:

- Exhaustion.
- Fever.
- Certain medications.
- Anxiety.
- Sudden noise.
- A full bladder.
- Excitement.

You shouldn't try to wake up a child who is having a night terror; just be there to comfort them when they do awaken.

## Sleepwalking

Also known as somnambulism, sleepwalking is reasonably common, with one in five children experiencing it at least once. It does not occur during REM stages, so it doesn't take place during the dreaming stage of sleep. Sleepwalking is when someone stands up, walks, or even carries out complex tasks while asleep.

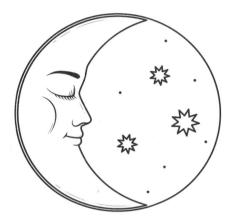

In extreme examples people have been known to leave the house and drive a car while sleepwalking!

A sleepwalker's eyes are usually open, and often they are capable of communicating, albeit they might not make much sense. A typical episode lasts around ten minutes, and the sleepwalker will usually not remember it the next morning. As with night terrors, you shouldn't try to wake a sleepwalker up—just make sure they are safe and be there to ensure they get back to bed safely afterward. Exact causes are not known, but in addition to the triggers mentioned above for night terrors, taking recreational drugs and an excess of alcohol can make an episode more likely.

## Some Other Sleep Disorders

Sleep disorders can reduce the number or quality of dreams a person has at night. People with the following disorders are thought to have more vivid nightmares than normal sleepers.

- **Sleep apnea**—Breathing stops for ten seconds or more during sleep.
- **Insomnia**—Trouble falling or staying asleep.
- **Narcolepsy**—Suddenly falling asleep at inappropriate times.
- **Sleep paralysis**—The feeling of being awake but not being able to move.

❋ ❋ ❋

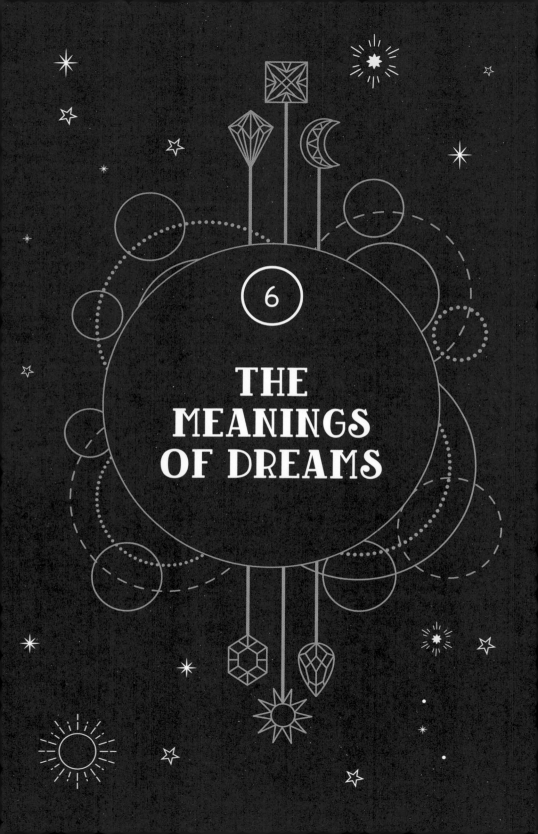

6

# THE MEANINGS OF DREAMS

We have looked at how we dream and what neurobiologists, psychologists, and religions say about dreaming. We have also seen how ancient civilizations and cultures viewed dreams, but what does it mean if we dream about all our teeth falling out? Should we cancel that vacation because we have had a couple of dreams in which a plane crashed into the sea?

While the content of some dreams can seem logical, taking place in a linear pattern, many dreams seem to be full of nonsensical motifs and items thrown together. But does a dream have to be logical to mean something, or is there meaning found in every dream?

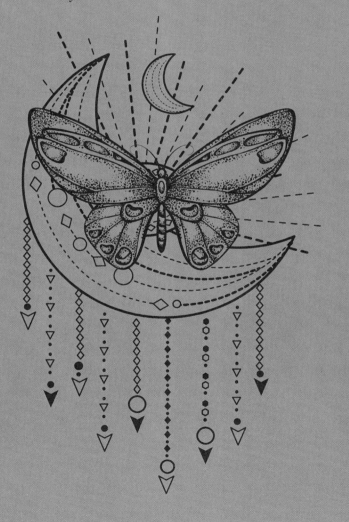

What follows are some of the most common dream themes and possible meanings for them based on the psychology behind the dreams and, in some cases, ancient mystical meanings and "old wives' tales" passed down through generations.

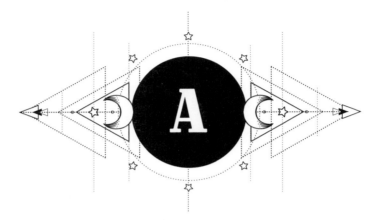

**Abandonment** To dream that you are abandoned suggests that it is time to leave behind past feelings and characteristics hindering your growth. Let go of your old attitudes. A more direct and literal interpretation of this dream is that you have a fear of being deserted, abandoned, or even betrayed. It may stem from a recent loss or a fear of losing a loved one. The fear of abandonment may manifest itself in your dream as part of the healing process and dealing with losing a loved one. It may also stem from unresolved feelings or problems from childhood. Alternatively, the dream indicates that you are feeling neglected or that your feelings are being overlooked. If you dream that you are abandoning someone else, it means that you are overwhelmed by the responsibilities you are taking on for other people.

**Abbey** An abbey is a religious complex of buildings in which monks live and worship. Thus, a dream about an abbey may be a metaphor for seeking spiritual guidance about a particular issue or developing your spiritual awareness in general.

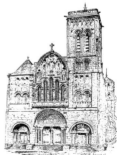

**Abdomen** Your abdomen in a dream refers to your instincts and repressed emotions. There is something in your real life that you "cannot stomach" or have difficulties accepting. You need to get it out of your system. Sometimes the dream symbol may be literal, and you may just be experiencing constipation or indigestion. If your abdomen is exposed in your dream, you have some trust issues and feel vulnerable. If the dream is about your swollen belly, it is a sign that there is a new project on the horizon.

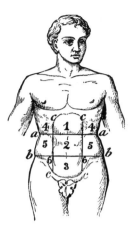

**Abduction** To dream about being abducted indicates that there are some circumstances or someone controlling or manipulating you. As a result, you lack control of your life and are feeling helpless.

**Abhorrence** If you dream that you hate someone, you likely have a strong dislike for that person in real life, and you are hiding some powerful feelings of resentment or aggression toward them that you don't think you can keep hidden for much longer.

**Abroad** Dreaming about being in a foreign country may indicate that you feel more adventurous of late and are willing to do or experience different things for a change.

**Abstinence** To dream that you practice abstinence from drinking, sex, or any other sensual temptation is a warning against being overconfident. Instead, it would help if you took things more slowly.

**Abuse** Dreams about abuse might link to past trauma, but they might also indicate you are in a relationship where someone else is dominating you—this might be in a work situation or a romantic relationship.

**Abyss** An abyss is symbolic of risk, and if one features in your dream, it means you are afraid of "taking the plunge." There is an obstacle that is in your way and causing you anxiety.

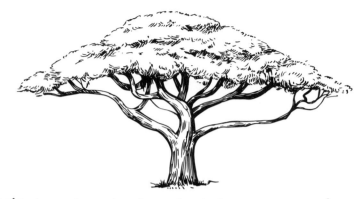

**Acacia** An acacia tree in a dream signals that you are aware of your mortality and have, perhaps, been thinking of your death.

**Accents** Hearing different accents in your dream might signify that you have difficulty communicating with someone in your conscious life or are struggling to understand someone and their needs.

**Accident** You may have made a mistake somewhere, and you are feeling guilty—perhaps you are punishing yourself for your error. However, there is also the possibility that dreaming about an accident is a warning that you need to slow down or take more care over something.

**Accordion** To hear the music of an accordion signifies some saddening and depressing matter. You need to focus on more joyous moments. To dream that you play the accordion denotes intense emotions that are causing physical strain to your body. You are feeling weary. Alternatively, the dream suggests that you need to work hard to achieve your goals.

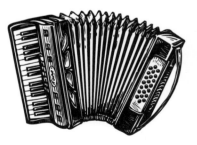

**Accused** Being accused of something you haven't done in real life can be frustrating and upsetting. However, if this is happening in your dream, it is likely to be a metaphor for being judged by someone else at the moment.

**Ace**  To see an ace from a deck of cards suggests ambiguity in your life and a need for clarity.

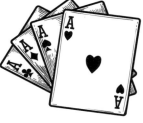

- The ace of hearts could mean that you are involved in a love affair.
- The ace of spades means that you are involved in a scandal.
- The ace of diamonds symbolizes your legacy or reputation.
- The ace of clubs suggests that you will be involved in some legal matter.

**Achievement**  Suppose you dream that you have achieved something. This indicates that you will be delighted with the outcome of a situation or project—the more significant the achievement, the greater the satisfaction.

**Acid**  Acid symbolizes toxicity, anger, revenge, and loss of control. If acid forms the main focus of your dreams, it is probably time to take a step back and examine your current emotions.

**Acorn**  Acorns symbolize strength and the ability to grow from something that was initially small. Perhaps you have some lofty ambitions that you need to focus on to ensure they are achieved.

**Actor or Actress**  Do you ever dream of being an actor on the stage or in a movie? If you do, then you must take care not to trust others too much because they may set out to deceive.

**Acupuncture**  If you dream that you are getting acupuncture, there is a possibility that you need healing—medically, spiritually, or emotionally. It would be best if you focus your energies on yourself.

**Addiction**  Are you dreaming of being addicted to alcohol or drugs? This is often symbolic of being an obsessive person, feeling overly dependent on a person, and believing that you can't cope without them.

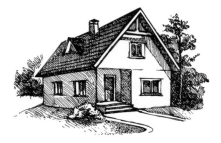

**Address** Do you ever dream of a previous house you owned? If you do, it is a sign that you need to look back to the past because something there could help you learn more about yourself. If you dream about a new address, you are more likely to be in the right frame of mind to change your environment.

**Admirer** A dream in which you have an admirer indicates that you are not showing your true positive qualities to others; it is as if they are only visible to one person—your admirer.

**Adopting** A dream in which you are adopting a child indicates that you are ready to take on something new—perhaps a new challenge or project.

**Adultery** If you commit adultery in a dream, it might be that your sexual desires are expressed as a need for attention from another person. If your partner is having the affair in your dream, you will likely feel insecure and unsettled and perhaps worried about being left alone.

**Adventure** Dreaming of going on an adventure indicates a current dissatisfaction with your life. Perhaps life is feeling too dull at the moment.

**Advice** Sometimes in a dream, a wise character will offer you words of advice, perhaps about your love life, family, or work. This is a message from your subconscious so it is useful to heed.

**Age** To dream of being old might indicate that you have some anxieties about growing older.

**Agoraphobia** When featured in a dream, the fear of open or crowded spaces may be a metaphor for social anxiety. Perhaps you are scared that people will judge you if you open up too much to them.

**Airplane**  A dream featuring an airplane means that an ambition has yet to be fulfilled.

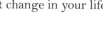

**Airport**  Airports are symbolic of arrivals and departures, and in a dream, this could indicate that you are on the brink of significant change in your life—usually in a good way.

**Ambulance**  An ambulance in a dream is said to warn that there will be some form of illness in the family.

**Amputation**  Losing a leg or an arm in a dream means that you could soon be suffering from slights and injustices.

**Angels**  Angels are generally perceived as being messengers of God who appear in your dreams to offer protection, guidance, and spiritual healing.

**Ants**  Ants symbolize action and industry, and a dream about them foretells a busy time ahead, with a lot of work to be done. Some people believe that dreams about insects predict several minor but irritating problems.

**Apocalypse**  To dream about an apocalyptic event is an indication that something potentially big and life-changing is about to happen—it could be positive or negative.

**Arguing**  A dream in which you are arguing with a member of your family or an ex-partner is often indicative of repressed emotions and unspoken grievances with that person. If you find yourself arguing with friends or family who are dead, this shows there are things you wish you had said to them when they were alive.

**Arrested**  Have you been arrested in your dream? Rather than suggesting that you have recently committed a crime, it is much more likely to signify that you are feeling restrained by something or someone, and it's time to try to get out from under their control.

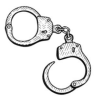

**Asthma**  There will be difficulties ahead is the warning of a dream about asthma.

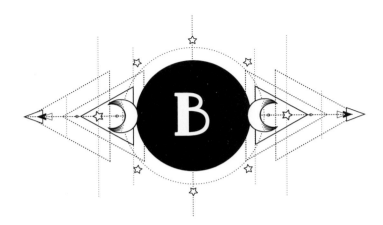

**Babies** Dreaming of babies does not mean that you are pregnant! Babies represent innocence, purity, helplessness, and new beginnings—perhaps these are qualities of your own that you don't usually show the world. Alternatively, a dream about a baby can foretell good luck for you and your family. This is a common dream that many people have from time to time.

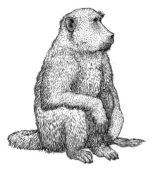

**Baboon** A baboon in your dream signifies that you need to be more expressive about something. You need to make your feelings more obvious to other people.

**Baby Clothes** Dreams about baby clothes are an indication that there are old habits and ways of behaving that you have now discarded.

**Baby Food** A dream that features baby food tells you that you need to nourish yourself and put yourself first for once. However, if you dream that you are fed baby food, you feel you are being taught something you already know in the real world.

**Baby Pram or Buggy** A dream featuring a baby pram can have a couple of meanings. On the one hand, it could symbolize your desire to start a family. On the other hand, if the pram is empty, you may be sad or have an unfulfilled goal.

**Baby Shower** A baby shower dream does not necessarily mean that you are pregnant. It is likely to mean that you are preparing to welcome something new into your life—of course, it could be a baby, but it could also be a new job, a new home, or a new hobby.

**Bachelor** Meeting a bachelor in your dream suggests that you are seeking freedom in your love life. For a man to dream that he is a bachelor indicates that he is having difficulty gaining his sense of self or sufficient freedom in a relationship. Alternatively, the bachelor could represent your masculine side and serve as a sign that you need to be less emotional.

**Back Door** A back door is symbolic of the need to search a little harder to find an answer to your problem. Sometimes the solution may not be obvious. Alternatively, the dream indicates that you are trying to find shortcuts.

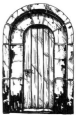

## BACK

If you dream about your back, it symbolizes your attitudes, strengths, burdens, and stance in the world.

- If your back is straight, then you are likely to be presenting a strong, confident self to the world, one with few worries.
- On the other hand, a hunched-over back signifies someone with many worries or burdens at the moment. It may relate to the stress and pressure that someone else is putting on you.
- If the back that you see in your dream is naked, you are likely to have secrets that you may have kept from others or aspects of yourself that you have kept hidden and shielded away. Also, consider the phrase "watch your back!"; this dream may be telling you to do just that.
- If the back you see is someone else's, consider this a warning that you should not lend money to anyone. In particular, lending money to friends will cause a rift in your relationship.
- To see a person turn their back on you signifies that you will be deeply hurt due to envy and jealousy.

**Backgammon**  Who doesn't like a good game of backgammon? To lose a game of backgammon symbolizes misfortune and a lack of luck in love. However, in a dream, a backgammon game is also likely to represent an unwelcome guest. You may be seeking the wrong type of person, making your path to love a difficult one.

**Backpack**  A full backpack in your dream is indicative of all the decisions, responsibilities, and stresses that you are carrying around at the moment. This is a time to see if you can relieve yourself of any of these. However, an empty backpack is symbolic of unknown adventures out there in the world waiting for you. It is time for you to take a risk and actively seek out those adventures.

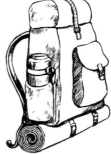

**Backpacking**  If your dream is about you being on a backpacking trip, you are likely to be really confident in yourself. You are independent, self-sufficient, and able to take care of yourself. You may well be reflecting on all the obstacles and problems that you have overcome to get to this point.

**Backward**  To dream that you are walking or moving backward indicates that your current course of action may be counterproductive. Whatever you are looking for in life seems to be moving away from you. Thus, you may feel a sense of failure or a belief that you cannot achieve your goals and aspirations. On the other hand, moving backward in your dream may indicate that you need to back off or retreat from a situation you are currently facing in your waking life.

**Bag**  A full bag represents prosperity, but an empty one foretells hard times ahead. If your dream is about you holding an expensive designer handbag, then you are being told to rein in your spending and extravagances and be a bit more prudent.

**Baggage**  To dream of carrying baggage and luggage indicates that you feel held back by problems and emotions and are "carrying the world on your shoulders." If, however, you dream of someone carrying your luggage for you, then it is a sign that you need to accept the help offered by others and not be too proud to admit that you need help.

**Bamboo** Bamboo is often seen as a metaphor for flexibility, strength, and survival under the harshest conditions. To dream about bamboo is indicative of the need for you to display these qualities right now due to an issue or situation in your conscious life.

**Bank** To dream about a bank is to be warned that there is the risk of money troubles that should not be ignored. Something needs to be sorted out quickly, so don't hesitate to make that important appointment with your accountant or banker.

**Barefoot** A dream about being barefoot can have a couple of different meanings. On the one hand, it could mean that you are exceptionally relaxed and carefree at the moment; but on the other hand, it may mean that you lack confidence and self-esteem. Some might even interpret a barefoot dream as representing poverty and shortage.

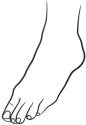

**Barking** Are you being grumpy at the moment and shouting at people more than usual? If so, this would be confirmed by you dreaming of dogs barking constantly. It's a sign to calm down and to work on whatever is making you angry. Did you know, however, that if you are deep in your REM sleep and there is very loud barking going on in the real world at the same time, you may end up unconsciously threading that noise into a dream about dogs or barking?

**Bats** Are you worried about dreaming of being surrounded by a colony of bats? No need to worry—bats symbolize rebirth, emerging as they do every evening at dusk. You may well be on the cusp of positive change or new opportunities.

**Beach** Lounging on a sandy beach is often many people's daydream, and to dream of a beach while asleep represents the same emotions and feelings—the need to relax and take things easy. Perhaps a vacation is long overdue.

# THE TOP TEN
# SYMBOLIC DREAMS

1. **Butterflies**. A dream focused on a butterfly is thought to be the most symbolic dream you can have. It suggests that you are about to undergo a spiritual transformation, after which nothing will be the same again. White butterflies are often thought to indicate that you can communicate with the dead.

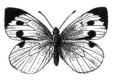

2. **Death**. Dreams about your death are likely to make you uncomfortable and perhaps scared that your demise is being foretold. This is not usually the meaning of such a dream. To dream of your own death is much more likely to indicate that it is time for you to let go of something or someone so that you can move forward spiritually and emotionally.

3. **Elephants**. Elephants are sacred in Buddhism and said to be the earthly manifestation of the Buddha himself. If an elephant features in your dream, it is a sign that you need to spend some time focusing on your spiritual awareness—maybe through yoga or meditation.

4. **Mother Nature**. Nature is constantly communicating with us, through a dramatic lightning storm, a wild wind, or even a sunny day. Often, we are too busy to stop and listen to the messages Mother Nature conveys to us. When this happens, we may dream about nature in some form—whether it be weather or a walk in the woods or climbing a granite outcrop. It is a subconscious message that we need to take the time to listen to Mother Nature and watch and feel nature as we go about our day.

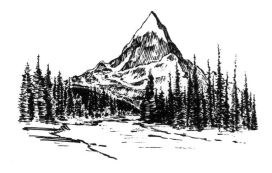

5. **Deities**. Divine figures such as Buddha, Jesus, or Muhammad emerging in your dreams are indications that you are currently undergoing a significant spiritual change—perhaps you had no spiritual belief originally and are now open to learning and embracing spiritual knowledge.

6. **Dolphins and Whales**. These beautiful creatures may appear in your dream in both a protective and a motivating way. They are letting you know that you should take a risk, go with your gut instinct, and do that thing you have been putting off, all with the assurance that everything will be okay.

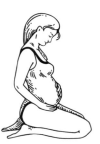

7. **Snakes.** Snakes are thought to represent rebirth, transformation, and healing. A significant, positive change is forecast for you if snakes emerge in your dream.

8. **Pregnancy**. Pregnancy dreams are often symbolic of a new birth in your life—not necessarily of a baby, but more likely of a new project, enterprise, or relationship.

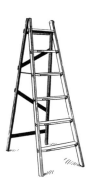

9. **Flying**. If you dream that you are flying above the world like Peter Pan, you are being encouraged to break free from any barriers holding you back. You are being told that you can have superpowers, if only you trust yourself to succeed.

10. **Ladders**. Ladders are considered ideal items for transcending the ordinary, everyday to a higher plane of consciousness. If you dream of ladders (or sometimes bridges or staircases), you are encouraged to take the steps to spiritual awareness and fulfillment.

**Beard** A beard represents the insight or wisdom that comes from age and experience. If you dream that you have a beard when you don't have one in real life, the dream means that you are trying to conceal your true feelings, and you are deceptive about some matter. Alternatively, the dream represents your attitude and says that you don't care what others think or say about you.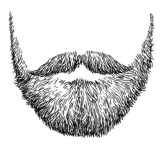
If you are a woman and dream of growing a beard, it signifies the masculine aspect of your personality, showing that you need to be more assertive and wield more power.

**Bed** A dream about a bed indicates that you should take time off for a well-deserved rest. If the bed is unmade, you must take care not to get into trouble.

**Bees** This is a common symbol that always means prosperity, progress, and praise for good work. Oddly enough, it can also warn of difficulties caused by a partner's parents.

**Bells** The bells ring out for good news to come, so keep an eye or an ear alert if bells appear in your dream.

**Birth** This is a common dream, and it means good luck, but it also indicates something new that is getting off the ground. However, it is common to dream about birth or labor if you are actually pregnant, reflecting your natural anxieties about the forthcoming event.

**Bouquet** While to receive a beautiful bouquet in your conscious life might be nice, to receive one in a dream means there will be a slight disappointment. Perhaps the warning is not to take things at face value and ask yourself what the motivation is behind the deed.

**Bread** Bread is an omen of good luck, enough to eat, and better times ahead. If you dream that you are feeding bread to ducks or other birds, the indication is that you are feeling particularly generous and thinking of others at the moment.

**Bridge** Think of the song "Bridge over Troubled Water," because if you see a bridge in your dream, it means that your troubles will soon pass. A bridge can also be a symbol that you are moving on and leaving any negativity behind.

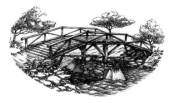

**Burial** This is not as scary or as negative as you might think: to dream of burial means that you will soon meet someone to love and to live with on a deep and meaningful basis.

**Burns** Rather than the pain that real-life burns can bring, dreaming of burns actually means that success is coming, and an end to troubles is on the horizon.

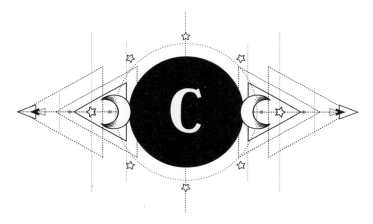

**Cab** If you are hailing a cab in your dream, there is a suggestion that you need to ask for help to be able to move forward, but if you are already riding in the cab, the indication is that you are being taken for a ride, that someone is taking advantage of you, and that you need to have a good think about who it might be.

**Cabbage** You might not eat cabbage in your waking life, but that doesn't mean you can't dream about it! If cabbage does turn up in a dream, it is a sign that you should not waste time with petty, insignificant things. Save your energy and focus on the important things in life.

**Cabinet** A cabinet symbolizes the female body and the womb, so it might be time to have a medical checkup if you are female. An alternative meaning is that you hide things from others and need to be more open with them.

**Cactus** The prickly spikes of a cactus appearing in your dream represent your boundaries being crossed, or they may mean that you cannot separate your private from your public life. Perhaps you are finding it difficult to separate work from your home life.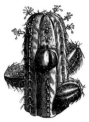

**Café** To dream that you are at a cafe represents your social life. The dream is telling you that it is time to call up old friends, to catch up and see what they are all doing.

**Cage** Dreaming of being in a cage has an obvious meaning of you being restrained, controlled, or trapped, by either a relationship or a situation. To dream of putting an animal in a cage has a more positive symbolism, which is that you will overcome your fears and succeed at whatever you decide to do. And if you dream of a bird in a cage? Well, that might have more to do with what you consider to be a lack of spirituality or a lack of ability to think freely, which, when you come to think of it, could also be due to someone else trying to hold you back.

**Cake** Realizing that you don't have to do everything yourself and share the load with friends and family might lead you to dream about cake. However, a half-eaten cake refers to missed chances or the failure to take advantage of specific opportunities.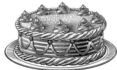

**Calculator** A dream in which a calculator features suggests that you need to think through a problem and carefully evaluate your options, and you need to lay out some sort of plan or outline. The symbol may also be a metaphor for someone who is calculating, cunning, and scheming.

**Calendar** To see a calendar in your dream represents the passing of time. This could make you feel anxious in your dream, especially if you are worried about aging. It may also be a reminder that there is something important coming up and a warning that you need to prepare for it.

**Calm**  Are you calm and collected in your dream? This could indicate that you are feeling happy and fulfilled in your waking life at the moment. If the dream is about someone telling you to calm down, this suggests that you are about to suffer some setback that would be worse if you can't control your emotions.

**Camel**  If your dream is about a camel, then the message you need to take on board is that you are currently doing too much and have too many burdens on your shoulders. It tells you that it is time to take a good look at your responsibilities, get rid of what you can, and delegate what you can, ensuring that you are left with only what you can manage.

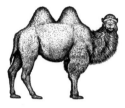

**Camera**  A camera in your dream signifies your desire to cling onto or to live in the past. Alternatively, it may indicate that you need to focus on a particular situation. Perhaps you need to get a clearer picture or idea. If the camera in your dream is broken, the indication is that you are ignoring an issue or refusing to see the big picture. To dream that you are on a hidden camera indicates that you feel that you are being scrutinized.

**Canary**  To see a canary in your dream represents happiness and harmony—you should take advantage of this and enjoy this period of your life. Alternatively, the dream could indicate your desires for a relationship or that a new relationship is blossoming.

**Candle**  A candle flame is often used in meditation to create a sense of peace, tranquility, and enlightenment, and within a dream, it fulfills the same purpose. An unlit candle, however, indicates disappointment and the failure to act; and if you are trying but failing to light the candle, you are likely to be grieving over a loss—of a person or an opportunity. A candle that is alight might also denote a birth in the family, while one that has been put out represents death in your circle.

**Cannibalism**  Is there something or someone in your life constantly draining your energy and overwhelming you? That might be why you are dreaming of cannibalism, which is representative of someone eating you alive!

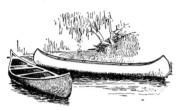

**Canoe** A canoe in your dream represents serenity, simplicity, and independence. It is also a reflection of your emotional balance. You are moving ahead via your power and determination.

**Cap and Gown** To wear a cap and gown in your dream indicates that you are transitioning to a higher level in your life. You are ready to move on to the next stage. To see someone in a cap and gown in your dream symbolizes your successes and accomplishments.

**Captive** Dreaming of being held captive or trapped somewhere has some obvious connections to feelings of entrapment in your conscious life—perhaps by a relationship, a job, or a financial situation.

**Car** To see yourself driving in your dream can symbolize being in control of your life and your emotions. For example, if you drive along a long, empty road, you are likely to feel very confident and willing to think big. However, if you are in your car, stuck in a traffic jam, you are likely to be feeling stuck and unable to negotiate your way around certain obstacles.

**Cat** There can be two interpretations of a cat dream: first, this indicates treachery around you, while another interpretation is of good luck, especially if the cat is black.

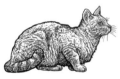

**Cemetery** Dreaming about a cemetery is, unfortunately, likely to indicate that you will hear of a death.

**Children Playing** The laughter and joy of children playing in your dream is an indication that happiness is on the way. It can also be a sign that you have been taking things too seriously of late and need to relax more.

**Clock** This is an indication of important business that requires attention. It is also a sign that there are important events on the way that you will need to monitor.

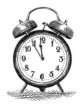

**Counting Money** Something worthwhile is on the way. It might not be a financial boost, but it will be good.

**Cow** Cattle refer to prosperity, because they relate to wealth in many traditions. It is generally accepted that it is very good luck for cattle to feature in your dream.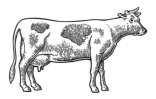

**Cradle** A baby's cradle is a metaphor for hopes and wishes to be fulfilled.

**Crossroads** A dream about a crossroads implies that you might be at a crossroads in your real life, where important decisions will soon become necessary.

**Crying Child** Although a crying child might be a negative thing or an annoyance in your conscious life, a crying child in your dream is an indication that a wish will be fulfilled. If you are deeply asleep, it is also possible that a child really is crying in the real world, and your subconscious is hearing it and winding it into your dream rather than waking you up!

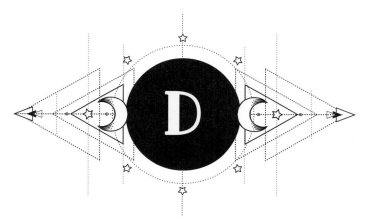

**Daffodils** One of the first signs of spring. A dream about daffodils usually means new beginnings, optimism, and the ability to start over again.

**Dahlias** These flowers in a dream are a sign of good luck—especially financially. Time to invest that money or perhaps buy that lottery ticket!

**Daisy** Daisies are all about love and friendship, so whether you are giving daisies to someone or receiving them, they signify a lasting and satisfying relationship.

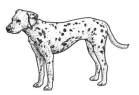

**Dalmatian**  To see a dalmatian in your dream suggests that you overlook your feelings in order to tend to the needs of others. You are a people pleaser.

**Damask Rose**  To see a damask rosebush in your dream signifies happy unions. If you receive a bouquet of damask roses in the dream, then you are about to experience true love.

**Dancing**  As you might imagine, dancing signifies freedom of movement and being happy. If you dream that you are dancing with a partner, you might be tapping into the intimacy and sensuality of the dance. However, if you are dancing with an ex-partner, it is more likely to signify that you are ready to let go and move on with no hard feelings.

**Dancing Child**  A dancing child in a dream points to difficulties ahead, for either you or someone close to you. Of course, the fact that the child is dancing means that the problems will be solved eventually and things will return to normal, but the problematic period is bound to happen.

**Dandelions**  Are you dreaming about blowing on the seeds of dandelions? This is often a throwback to childhood, especially if your childhood was happy and carefree. However, such a dream may mean that you are trying to regain that feeling of youth and freedom and that you are worried about time speeding by.

**Dandruff**  To dream that you have dandruff indicates that you are misusing your energy. You may have been under a lot of stress and tension. You should rethink the way you are approaching any of your current problems. Alternatively, this dream may suggest a lack of self-esteem.

**Danger**  Dreaming about being in danger or at risk from something is often an indication that you need to be cautious about something or someone in your conscious life. Perhaps you are taking too many chances at the moment with your feelings, your safety, or your money.

**Darkness** Darkness is often associated with negative symbols such as evil, death, and fear. If, however, you feel safe in your dream about the dark, then you are likely to be happy to "be in the dark" about something and satisfied with not knowing all the ins and outs of a situation. To be lost in the dark might indicate that you are feeling depressed or down at the moment and can't see a way out of your situation.

**Dartboard or Darts** If you see a dartboard in your dream, there is an indication that you are feeling hostility from someone and that you need to express your anger and feelings more directly. Alternatively, the dartboard may symbolize one of your goals. You need to try to take a shot 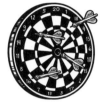 at something new and overcome your fear of failure. To dream that you are throwing darts in your dream refers to some hurtful or harmful remarks that you have made or that someone else has said about you.

# DATE

A dream about being on a date represents your need for self-discovery and self-awareness. You are getting to know some hidden aspects of yourself and acknowledging your hidden talents.

- It may reflect your anxieties about dating or finding acceptance.
- The dream may be a "rehearsal" for an actual date you may be going on, as the dream serves to overcome anxieties you may have.
- Are you being greedy and dating two people in your dream? This signifies passion in your personal relationship. This dream does not necessarily mean that you want to stray from your significant other, but it may denote some anxiety about some major change that is happening within the relationship.
- You might dream of a specific date, as in a particular month, day, and year, and this represents the passing of time and perhaps a recollection of past events.
- The dream may also be a reminder of a special event, appointment, or important date ahead of you in your everyday life.
- Also, consider the significance of the numbers in the date.

**Daughter**  To see your daughter in your dream represents your waking relationship with your daughter and the qualities she projects. If the relationship in the dream is warm and close, then that reflects your real-life relationship. If, however, things are strained and distant in your waking relationship, this is likely also to be reflected in your dream. If you do not have a daughter, it symbolizes the feminine aspect within yourself and the need to express it.

**Daughter-in-Law**  If you see your daughter-in-law in your dream, this is a signal that an unusual and unexpected incident will give you either much happiness or much distress, depending on her demeanor in your dream.

**Dawn**  Dawn is a symbol of rejuvenation, enlightenment, and vitality. You are emerging from one stage in life and have a new understanding or a new start going on in your life.

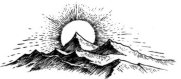

**Day**  A sunny day symbolizes clarity or positivity and implies that you are currently seeing things clearly. If the day is cloudier or gloomy, then sadness or a period of depression is indicated. A stormy day is symbolic of a change that will wipe the slate clean, sort out problems that have been hanging about, and clear the decks for your next project.

**Dead End**  To dream that you have come to a dead end might have a literal meaning: you have come to the end of something—a project or a relationship, maybe. However, it is also an indication that something is no longer working and that you need to find an alternative way of achieving a goal.

**Dead People**  Dreaming of dead people is not as scary or as harmful as you might think. If the person is recently deceased and a close family member or friend, the dream might be your subconscious helping you keep them "alive" and fresh in your mind. The dream may also be allowing you to clear up some unfinished business with the deceased, perhaps an unresolved argument. It is not uncommon for someone to dream regularly about a recently deceased person, and the dreams can be used to come to terms with what has happened. The dead may have other functions to play in your dreams—sometimes they are there to reassure you that you are doing all right, while at other times they might be giving advice and guidance.

**Deadline** With constant deadlines in our conscious world, it is not unusual for us to dream about deadlines or ticking clocks. Such dreams indicate that we are preoccupied with time and time running out, and that we need to slow down and prioritize the important things in life.

**Deaf** If you are not deaf in real life, if you dream that you are deaf, you feel unheard and sidelined over something important to you. You cannot communicate your frustration and hurt to someone, and it is making your frustration worse. On the other hand, such a dream can point out that you are unwilling to hear something that others are saying now, and perhaps you are reluctant to acknowledge the truth of something.

**Death** Some people dream about the death of someone who is very much still alive in the conscious world. Such a dream can be uncomfortable, especially if the person is someone close to you. It doesn't mean that that person will die in real life, but it might mean that something is missing in your relationship with that person, and perhaps something needs to be resolved to save it. It can be frightening to experience your own near-death experience while dreaming, but this is thought to show that you are being given a second chance at something, which of course is not at all frightening. To dream that 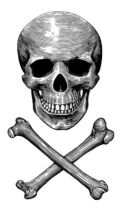 you actually die can also be framed positively because it can mean that you are on the brink of a transformation and that a significant change is about to happen, often in a spiritual sense.

**Debate** To dream that you are in a debate symbolizes the inner turmoil or conflict that you are experiencing. However, it also means that you will find closure to those unresolved issues.

**Debt** A dream about debt can mean that you have some financial worries at the moment. The unconscious stress and anxiety have probably caused such a dream that being in debt causes. It can, however, also signify imbalance, struggle, worry, and trouble in some personal situation or business matter. Another interpretation is that you are putting too many demands on others, and you are actually in debt to them in terms of time and goodwill.

**Decapitation** To dream that you are decapitated indicates that you are not thinking clearly and are refusing to see the truth. You need to confront the situation or the person despite the pain and discomfort you might feel in doing so. The dream also suggests that you tend to act before you think.

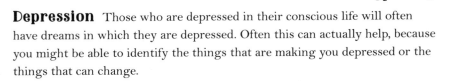

**Deer** A deer is said to symbolize natural beauty, majesty, and gentleness, but also alertness. These are all qualities that you might need to focus on in your conscious life.

**Depression** Those who are depressed in their conscious life will often have dreams in which they are depressed. Often this can actually help, because you might be able to identify the things that are making you depressed or the things that can change.

**Desert** If you dream that you are walking through a desert, you may feel lonely or isolated in your conscious life.

**Doctor** A doctor is obviously symbolic of ill health, so to dream of one warns that illness is on the way for either you or someone close to you.

**Dog** A dog is a symbol of loyalty, so if you have doubted someone's sincerity, it seems that they are trustworthy after all. Unfortunately, sometimes the dog dream means malicious gossip, especially by associates at your place of work.

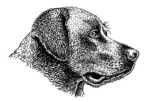

**Dove** Traditionally doves are a metaphor for peace and happiness, and a dream about doves indicates that these are coming your way. It also means happiness in love.

**Drowning** To dream that you are drowning is indicative that there are difficulties ahead that make planning useless.

**Dungeon** A dungeon is symbolic of danger and darkness, either for you or for those around you.

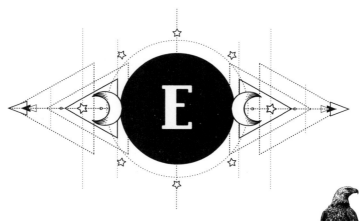

**Eagles** Eagles symbolize nobility, courage, and pride. To see one in your dream may indicate that you are struggling heroically to reach your goals.

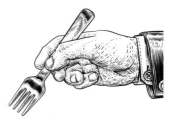

**Earth** A dream that features the earth is telling you that you need to be more grounded and rational. But, on the other hand, if the ground opens up, as in an earthquake, it may indicate a project or a relationship situation that is wrong for you and which you are afraid of joining.

**Eating** Eating with other people symbolizes friendship and intimacy; to dream about eating alone can signify loneliness and even loss.

**Elevator** An elevator symbolizes a rise in stature, career, money, or consciousness.

**Emergency** If your dream features some kind of emergency, you are being warned that something needs your attention in your conscious life.

**Emotions** Emotional dreams provide you with a safe outlet for any pent-up emotions that you are afraid to express in your conscious life.

**Empress or Emperor** An empress or emperor in a dream warns that pride will cause a fall to someone close to you.

**End**  To dream of an end to something could signify that you have come to an end to something in your conscious life—perhaps a project has ended or a goal has been reached.

**Exile**  Have you dreamed that you have been exiled? This could mean the loss of something or someone valuable or that you are kept in the dark about something.

## COVID-19 AND DREAMS

Since the worldwide breakout of the COVID-19 pandemic, many people have claimed that the virus has affected their dreams. There have been so many claims that an expert team from the University of Helsinki conducted dream research on 4,000 sleepers. More than half of the participants stated that their sleep patterns had worsened since the pandemic and that the number of vivid dreams had increased. Most COVID-related dreams were about anxiety and worry about catching the virus and the dangers of people not social distancing or wearing masks. In addition, a survey in the journal *Frontiers of Psychology* reported a 26 percent increase in people saying they had nightmares since the outbreak started.

Some of the dreams people have been having are so vivid or disturbing that thousands of people are logging their nightmares on the Internet (see www.idreamofcovid.com, for example).

It isn't just fear and anxiety of the pandemic that has caused people to have vivid dreams. Some are reporting nightmares and disturbing dreams after having had a vaccine dose. It is important to note that nightmares and bad dreams are not recorded side effects of any currently available vaccines.

Scientists have been quick to reassure people that having a vivid dream after a vaccine injection is perfectly normal and that the reaction is short-lived. It is thought to be caused by a combination of anxiety about possible side effects of the vaccine and the fact that sleep (and in particular REM sleep) is disturbed by the body having to make antibodies as a response to the vaccine.

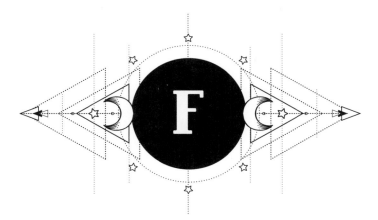

**Failure**  You might dream of failure if you feel insecure and worthless at the moment. Maybe you are overwhelmed or feeling under pressure to succeed at something.

**Falling**  Dreams about falling from a great height are widespread. While some dream interpreters might dramatize things by claiming that if you hit the ground in your dream, you will die in real life, the reality is that dreaming about falling is much more likely to indicate that you are worried about something. Perhaps you are concerned about failing at something in your work life or your love life, or it could mean that you need to rethink something.

**Family**  If your own family makes an appearance in your dream, it is most likely to indicate that you feel secure and loved. However, if it becomes a recurring dream, it could mean that you are overdependent on your family and need to stand on your own two feet a bit more.

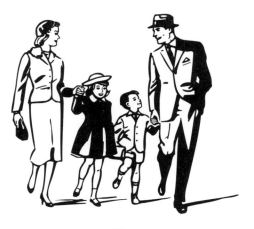

# WHY DO I STILL DREAM
# ABOUT MY EX?

It is common to dream about an ex–romantic partner. It doesn't seem to matter how long ago you split up, or how long it has been since you have seen them, whether you finished on good terms or not, or who was responsible for the split, or even if you are now happily married to someone else and have four children!

There is a range of ways in which your ex might turn up in your dream:

- **Sex with the ex**—Dreaming about having sex with your ex does not necessarily mean that you want to have sex with them! On the one hand, it could mean that you are missing some part of your previous sexual relationship and that your current sex life is not as good as it should be. On the other hand, perhaps sex with your ex wasn't that good, and subconsciously you would like the opportunity to go back and improve it.

- **Fighting with the ex**—Dreaming about fighting and arguing with your ex-boyfriend or ex-girlfriend can mean that you are still carrying some unresolved anger at them. Perhaps you didn't have the chance to get it all off your chest and tell them what you thought of them in real life. Conversely, dreaming about fighting with your ex may be symbolic of the way you feel in a current relationship. Perhaps you have fears and worries about your current relationship or feel unable to communicate freely with your current partner. You may be expressing these feelings in your dream by directing them at an ex.

- **A dying, dead, or sick ex**—Don't worry, this type of dream rarely actually means that your ex is dying, dead, or ill! It is more likely to point to unresolved issues and too many things that have been left unsaid in your previous relationship. Perhaps you are filled with regret that you won't have the chance to let them know just how badly they hurt you or how much you missed them, or even how much you loved them. However, such a dream does not have to be negative; it can symbolize the end of an era and the beginning of a new one. It may mean that you can finally put your memories and emotions from that relationship away and focus now on a new relationship.

- **Getting back with the ex**—This dream can be uncomfortable to wake up from, and it might make you feel out of sorts all day. It doesn't actually signify that you want to get back with your ex-partner, but it may be that you are single at the moment or in an unsatisfactory relationship; therefore, dreaming about reconciling with your ex is likely to have you thinking of the things about a relationship that you like and need and are lacking at the moment. On the other hand, the significance of the dream could be that you see history repeat itself at the moment. Perhaps you are making the same mistakes with your new partner that you did with your ex, or maybe you are letting your current partner treat you in the same negative way as your ex did. The dream could act as a warning that you need to change something.

- **The helpful ex**—Have you dreamed that your ex is helping you out somehow, perhaps by giving you advice? One interpretation of such a dream could be telling you not to make the same mistakes you did in the past, or not to accept the exact behavior you did from them from a new partner. It doesn't matter what the help or advice is that your ex is giving in the dream—it is just a metaphor or reminder that you need to learn from the past.

- **The cheating ex**—This is quite a common dream. It doesn't matter whether your ex really did cheat on you, but it indicates that you are currently worried about being betrayed by someone in your current world. This might be a betrayal by a friend or by a new partner, which may mean cheating with someone else, business fraud, or some other stab in the back.

- **Bumping into the ex**—Dreaming of casually seeing your ex, perhaps in a shop or at a party, is indicative that there are qualities that you miss about them. It could be that they are not in your life at all now, and you miss their presence, although not necessarily romantically.

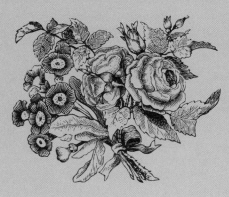

**Father**  A father figure may symbolize authority and protection, but it depends on what your conscious relationship is like with him. If you have a tense or distant relationship, having your father show up in your dream might imply that you need to make an effort to get to know him better or develop a better relationship. If your father is angry at you in your dream, it may be a sign that you are doing something in your conscious life of which he would disapprove.

**Fear**  A dream in which you are fearful could symbolize your current anxiety about something in your conscious life. Perhaps you are unsure that you have made the right decision about something or are unsure whether you are doing something correctly.

**Feet**  Feet represent mobility, freedom, and stability, so dreaming about your own feet might refer to the need for you to ground yourself or move on. Obviously, you would need to decide which option is right for you. If it is other people's feet that you are dreaming about, you are probably overly concerned about where they are going 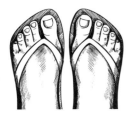 and what they are doing, so perhaps it is time for you to focus on yourself and your direction of travel. Feet are often seen as a metaphor for prosperity, and to dream about feet is to welcome some luck and prosperity into your life.

**Finding Money**  Finding money in your dream is not as lucky as it might be in the real world! It is likely to mean that you must guard against losses.

**Fighting**  A dream fight symbolizes inner turmoil and self-conflict.

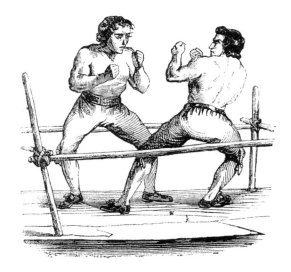

# FOOD AND DREAMS

Many people say that after eating certain foods or delicacies, or after having drunk a specific drink, they experience nightmares, and cheese seems to be the main culprit. However, does cheese really give you nightmares, or is this an urban myth?

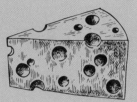

The British Cheese Board (yes, really!) was so intrigued that it decided to conduct some research. During a week-long experiment, 200 participants were given twenty grams of cheese thirty minutes before going to sleep. Expecting to hear stories of strange dreams and nightmares, the researchers asked each participant to keep a sleep log. Surprisingly, none of the participants reported experiencing a nightmare, and 75 percent of them recorded a series of good, restful nights of sleep throughout the week.

What the British Cheese Board research did discover, however, was that different cheeses led to different types of dreams:

- Cheddar: fame.
- Lancashire: work.
- Red Leicester: childhood.
- Cheshire: no dreams.
- Stilton: bizarre dreams.

Why do some people report nightmares after eating cheese and others have a perfect night's sleep, and even others claim that they had the best night's sleep for ages? Well, it's all about the nutrients. Cheese is an excellent source of an amino acid called tryptophan, which reduces stress and encourages peaceful sleep. However, cheese also contains a high level of vitamin B6, and this vitamin can increase the level of serotonin, which can cause dreams to be more vivid and memorable.

Of course, it's not all about cheese. There are also stories about caffeine in coffee, melatonin in bananas, spices in curry and hot sauces, and sugar in carbonated drinks, cookies, and ice cream, all of which are said to be the cause of vivid dreams, nightmares, and disturbed sleep. But some foods have the opposite effect, leading to a stress-free night of deep and comforting sleep. Foods such as peanut butter and jelly (jam to our British readers), almonds, kiwi, turkey, or chamomile tea are excellent alternatives.

## FLYING

Dreaming that you are flying, perhaps soaring above your day-to-day life and home, can be positive or negative. On the one hand, flying dreams might make you feel free and liberated, carefree and without worry; on the other hand, a flying dream might be more indicative of a need to get away from the realities of everyday life. Those who feel socially constrained may be more likely to dream about flying, illustrating a need to break free from mainstream values. Another possibility is that a flying dream indicates the need to break or cut ties with someone or somewhere.

### SOUL FLIGHT

Dreams of flying can be part of an out-of-body experience, in which the soul or spirit of the person takes a trip and returns to the sleeping body later.

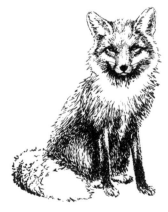

**Fox** One interpretation is that plans succeed beyond your expectations, while another is to watch out for sly people and back-stabbers.

**Friend** To dream about a friend, especially a close one, indicates that good luck and happiness are on the way.

**Friend in Trouble** Either a friend will need help from you or vice versa.

**Friend's House** If your dream is set in a friend's house, there will be good luck in work and with plans in general.

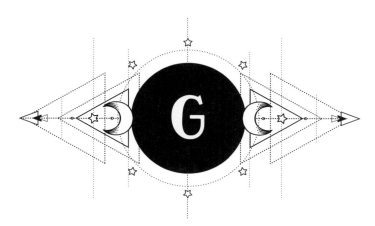

**Gagging** Dreaming that you are gagging or choking indicates that you are trying but failing to say something to someone. Perhaps you are not genuinely communicating the way that you feel about a situation.

**Gambling** Gambling in a dream symbolizes risk-taking and impulsiveness. If you are an actual gambler in your conscious life, this might be a warning to start being more risk-averse. On the other hand, if you are generally not a gambler, this type of dream may suggest that you take a chance and be a little more spontaneous with something or someone.

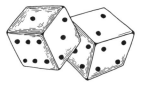

**Gang** If you dream that you are confronted by a gang, you may be feeling pressured or intimidated by a group of people in your conscious life. To dream that you are actually a member of a gang could mean that you have been a little heavy-handed in your dealings with someone recently.

**Garden** A garden with evergreens and flowers means excellent peace of mind and comfort. Women who see a lovely garden will be famous and happy in their family life, while walking through a lover's garden brings happiness and the kind of money that will make the woman independent. A vegetable garden means loss, misery, and loss of reputation.

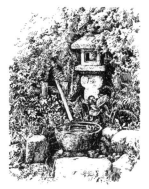

**Garden of Eden**  The garden of Eden symbolizes peace, harmony, beauty, and tranquility—emotions that you may be seeking at the moment.

**Garlic**  A garlic patch suggests a rise from poverty to wealth. A woman will partner with someone who will give her a good standard of living and not look for love. Eating garlic means taking a realistic view of life.

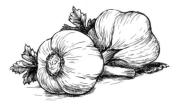

**Gate**  To see an open gate in your dream and to walk through it indicates that you are entering a new phase of life. A closed gate hints that you are not ready or willing to move on yet.

**Gems**  Dreaming of gems foretells happiness in love and in your career or business.

**Ghost**  There are several possible meanings to seeing a ghost in your dream. For example, if the ghost is of someone currently living, you should treat it as a warning that person means you harm. If the ghost is yourself, you may be afraid of death or dying. To see the ghost of a family member or friend who has died indicates that there are some regrets about your relationship with that person. Finally, if you dream that you are being haunted by a ghost, you are likely to be refusing to acknowledge something from your past.

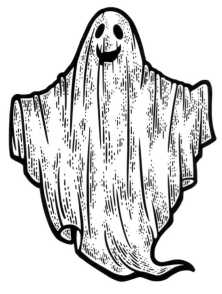

**Giant**  A giant in your dream signifies a huge obstacle stopping you from achieving something. The dream shows that you need to think of ways to reduce the challenges in your way.

# GLASS

Looking through glass shows that what you are hoping for will not work out and you may be very disappointed.

- Seeing your own image in a mirror predicts taking up with a partner who is neglectful and unfaithful, and investments that are a waste of money.
- Seeing someone else's face in a mirror suggests that you are leading a double life, and that you are setting out to deceive others.
- Breaking a mirror is generally seen as a bad omen.
- A full drinking glass means that you will soon hear from a loved one, but if it is empty, there will be temporary difficulties, and a broken glass means wishes will come true.
- A married woman seeing her husband in a mirror is a warning to keep an eye on him in case he starts to look at someone else.
- If a married man dreams of seeing a woman whom he doesn't know in a mirror, he may lose money in some get-rich-quick scheme.
- Looking through a glass window means you will soon find work or change to a better job, but you will have to work hard.

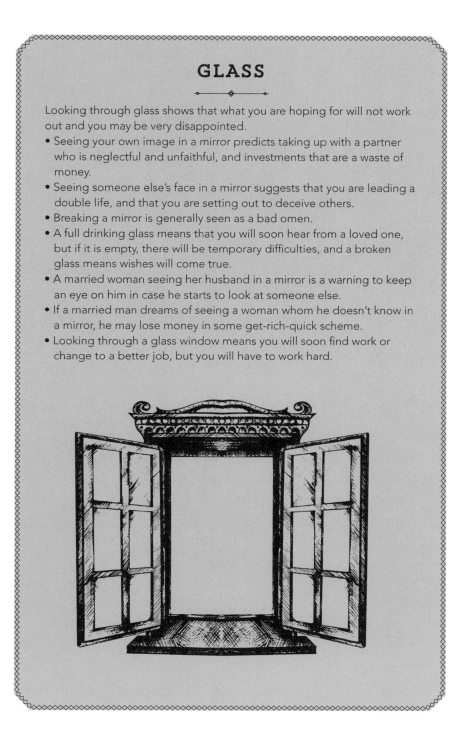

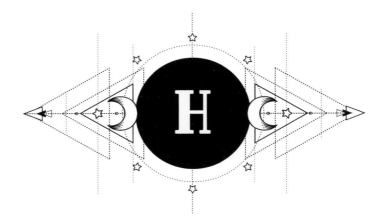

**Hair** Hair is often a sign of virility, strength, and attractiveness, so to dream that you are losing your hair shows that you are worried about losing some part of your personality. If another person is cutting your hair, it could reflect a concern that someone in your conscious life is holding a grudge against you. Alternatively, you might dream that your hair won't stop growing, and this is often a sign of feeling overwhelmed about something and of having too many things to cope with.

**Hand** You will be surrounded by flatterers.

**Hawk** A dead hawk indicates that something is being hidden from you, and maybe someone is being disloyal or talking about you behind your back. Conversely, a majestic, flying hawk is symbolic of you being very perceptive and able to look at a situation from the outside.

**Hazard** Perhaps a little bit obvious, but dreaming about hazards is often an indication that there are obstacles and hazards in your way in the conscious world that you need to navigate and remove.

**Hearse** To see a hearse in a dream does not mean that someone is going to die and you are going to attend a funeral. Its appearance in your dream suggests that you are currently in a transformative time in your life, where you are moving on from the end of something and are getting ready to embrace the new.

**Horse**  A black horse denotes disappointments, while a brown one suggests stagnation and delays. A gray horse indicates restlessness and uncertainty, and a white horse foretells financial progress.

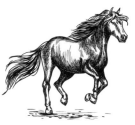

**Horseshoe**  A horseshoe in your dream means a pleasant journey is to come in the near future.

**House**  This is an important dream, because it shows the state of your mind and the things that are most worrying. If the house is a mess, it shows confusion in your life, while a house full of people shows that things are getting out of your control.

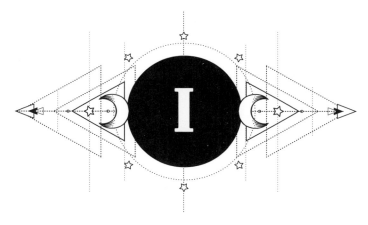

**Ice**  Nothing seems to flow at the moment, and that might be the reason for dreaming about frozen ice. Alternatively, it could be a warning to be careful about something.

**Iceberg**  We all know that there is so much more to an iceberg than just that which we see on the surface. Dreaming of an iceberg is symbolic of the need for you to dig deeper with regard to an issue and not take things at face value.

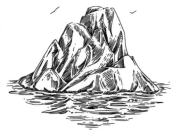

**Ignoring Someone** This might reflect a real-life scenario in which you are currently annoyed with someone and ignoring them. If so, the function of the dream would be for you to consider whether it might be better just to have it out with them. Alternatively, to dream about ignoring someone can indicate that you are willfully ignoring something negative about their personality or behavior.

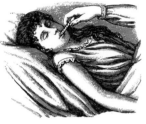

**Illness** Dreaming about illness, which may be yours or someone else's, does not automatically mean that anyone is ill. It is more likely to be a nudge for you to start enjoying life and a reminder that life is short.

**Imprisonment** Are you feeling trapped? Are people stopping you from making decisions for yourself? Feel like someone is oppressively interested in what you are doing? Being micromanaged at work? These are all reasons why you might dream about being imprisoned. It can also be a warning not to get into something that you would regret, but it can also mean delays and problems that will take time to sort out.

**Indecision** The obvious interpretation of dreaming about being indecisive is that you *are* indecisive in your conscious world. Perhaps there is a big decision that you are being asked to make that is going to have a big impact on your life and that of others. This type of dream is urging you to take your time over the decision and not rush into anything.

**Infestation** To dream of an infestation of insects or rats can have two meanings. On the one hand, you may feel that a small issue has been blown out of proportion and is now taking over your life; on the other hand, you may feel that your privacy is being invaded by someone or something, and it is time to keep your own counsel.

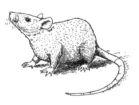

**Infidelity** Feelings of insecurity or dissatisfaction with a current relationship may cause you to dream of infidelity—either yours or your partner's.

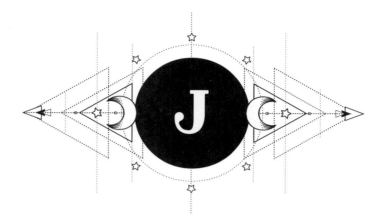

**Jar** An empty jar denotes a shortage of money and unhappiness, but a full jar means success. If you buy a jar in a shop, you will be successful but only after a great deal of hard work. Broken jars indicate health worries or other disappointments.

**Jaundice** Dreaming of having jaundice denotes prosperity after a temporary setback. Seeing others with jaundice means untrustworthy friends and prospects that won't have a good outcome.

**Job** To dream about your current job is an indication that you have a lot going on at the moment at work. Perhaps you are in the middle of a difficult project or you're working to tight deadlines. If the dream is about looking for a new job, it is likely to mean that you are dissatisfied with some aspect of your current life and looking for more excitement. Losing a job in your dream is pointing to the insecurity that you might be feeling about your current job.

**Journey** "Life is a journey," or so they say, and the obvious meaning of a dream about a journey is that it is a metaphor for your conscious life. Maybe you are embarking on a journey of discovery. A journey also implies leaving something or some place, which you need to do if you are to fully embrace the future.

**Jumping** Jumping off a cliff into the ocean below is symbolic of taking a risk and going for it. If you land safely in the ocean in your dream, the advice would be to take that risk. An unhappy ending to such a jump might suggest that you need to take some more time to consider all the pros and cons before taking the chance.

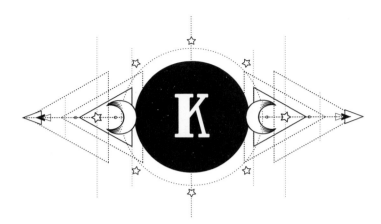

**Kangaroo** Seeing a kangaroo shows you will outwit someone who is trying to put you in a bad position and ruin your reputation. If a kangaroo attacks you, your reputation will definitely be in jeopardy. If you kill a kangaroo, you will overcome obstacles and succeed despite the activities of enemies.

**Kettle** Seeing kettles in a dream suggests that you have a lot of work ahead of you, and it will be heavy going. A boiling kettle is a good omen as it shows things will soon change for the better. A broken kettle suggests failure and a letdown. The color of the kettle is important, because if it is light, your future will be easy and pleasant, but if it is black, there will be a disappointment in love.

**Key** A key can be a symbol of many different things. Perhaps it is referring to a house move or even a move to another part of the country. It might be a metaphor for finally discovering the truth about something or someone. If you dream of using the key to lock a safe or a desk drawer or a door, the implication could be that you are keeping things too close to your chest and need to be more open with others. Dreaming of finding a key indicates that you are on the verge of discovering the answer to a problem.

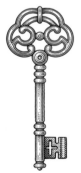

**Killing** Have you been short-tempered and irritated with someone recently? If so, you may well dream about killing them! Don't worry; it doesn't mean that you are really likely to murder anyone. It is more likely to be a suggestion that you take a breath and work out exactly what the issue is with the other person and then talk it through with them. If you are being killed in your dream, you are likely to be feeling overwhelmed and unappreciated.

**Kingfisher** Calmness, dignity, and majesty are three words conjured up by the image of a kingfisher—all qualities that you might need to demonstrate when things get difficult.

**Kiss** A kiss symbolizes love, affection, harmony, and romance—emotions you might be yearning for at the moment.

**Knife** A dream involving a knife is a warning of danger.

**L**

**Lake** Seeing a lake in your dream has a lot of relevance to your present state of mind. For instance, is the lake smooth and tranquil, or is it choppy and disturbed? Can you see the edges of the lake, or does it extend forever into the distance, meaning that you can't cope with the size and scope of an issue, or maybe the problem is too difficult to handle?

**Lamp** If the lamp is lighted, it is a good omen for business affairs, but if it has been turned off, someone is keeping something from you.

**Lawyer**  A dream involving a lawyer or solicitor is a warning of legal or financial difficulties.

**Leaving**  If the dream is about you leaving a place or someone, it's a metaphor for an end to something and an indication that it is time to move on. If you dream that someone is leaving you, then you are most likely feeling insecure about something in your conscious life.

**Lion**  Lions are symbolic of independence, leadership, and boldness. To dream of a lion is an indication that you will soon take the lead in an important enterprise.

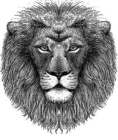

**Losing Money**  This is not as bad as you might think, because it is likely to mean that plans will succeed beyond your wildest hopes.

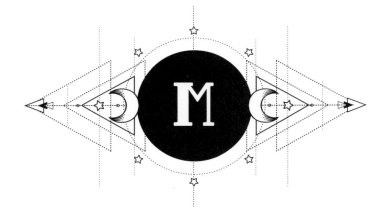

**Macaroni**  Macaroni or any small pasta might foretell small losses, but large amounts of such pasta show that you can save money if you take care. This is also a classic omen of a tall, dark stranger entering a woman's life—but whether he will be any good or not... well, time will tell!

**Maggots**  Maggots often symbolize anxiety and fear about death, either your own or that of someone close to you. Black maggots indicate that you are in denial about a problem, and maggots coming out of your mouth suggest that you have not been honest about something that you have said or done recently.

# MEDICATION AND DREAMS

Medications that influence the neurotransmitters in our brains, such as antidepressants and blood pressure medicines, can cause disturbing dreams and nightmares for some users. Some particular drugs are especially known for this:

- **Antidepressants.** Also known as SSRIs, or selective serotonin reuptake inhibitors, some types of antidepressants have the known side effect of inducing vivid and disturbing dreams. Particular culprits are Prozac (fluoxetine), Zoloft, Paxil, and vilazodone.
- **Blood pressure medications.** Beta-blockers, used to regulate blood pressure and slow the heart in the case of atrial fibrillation or angina, are the biggest medicinal cause of nightmares and vivid dreams. Bisoprolol, propranolol, metoprolol, atenolol, and labetalol are all types of beta-blockers for which this is a common side effect.
- **Antihistamines.** Over-the-counter anti-allergy tablets are regularly blamed for causing bad dreams, in particular Benadryl, Zyrtec, Claritin, Allegra, and Aller-Chlor.
- **Steroids.** The steroids prednisone and methylprednisone can affect brain chemistry, mood, and quality of sleep, thus causing vivid and disturbing dreams.
- **Medication for Parkinson's disease.** Amantadine is a common drug used to help treat some of the symptoms of Parkinson's disease. Some of its reported side effects include confusion, insomnia, hallucinations, and vivid dreams, often of a sexual nature.
- **Statins.** Cholesterol-lowering statins can cause dreams and disturbed sleep in some patients.
- **Medication for Alzheimer's.** Donepezil and rivastigmine are two drugs used to treat dementia in Alzheimer's patients that, unfortunately, can cause nightmares if taken at night.

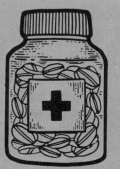

It should, of course, be noted that these medications have many beneficial qualities for those who need them; some are lifesaving. That they can cause disturbed sleep, bad dreams, or nightmares should not be a reason to stop taking them.

**Magpie**  Dreaming of a magpie shows the possibility of a quarrel to come. This is also a warning to be careful of what you say and whom you say it to.

**Manuscript**  Dreaming of writing a manuscript refers to your ambitions, goals, and desires. You are perhaps too anxious to achieve a goal, so you need to slow down and enjoy the process.

**Map**  Dreaming about a map means that you will take a long journey for work or for pleasure. There is also the possibility of taking part in a great adventure.

**Mice**  Mice, hamsters, chipmunks, gerbils, and small animals, in general, indicate a number of minor troubles and nuisances to come.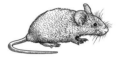

**Mirror**  If a mirror features heavily in your dream, there are two possible meanings. On one hand, it may indicate that it is time for you to take a good, honest look at your behavior in recent months. Is there anything you are ashamed of? On the other hand, it could indicate that you should expect some flattery from the opposite sex in the near future.

**Mistletoe**  We all know that we should kiss under the mistletoe and, appropriately, a dream about mistletoe indicates that good relationships are coming.

**Moon**  The moon suggests that you can't see things clearly and that deception may be in the air. The advice here is to wait for things to be revealed before acting.

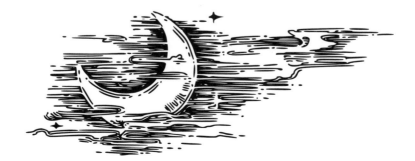

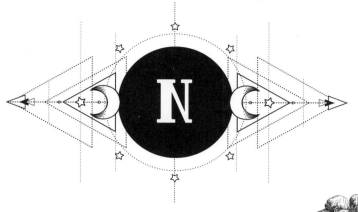

**Naked** Dreaming about being naked is very common. It shows that you are insecure about something or worried about revealing inefficiency or imperfections. "Imposter syndrome"—the persistent thought that your success is not deserved or has not been achieved through your own skills and efforts—is a common cause of dreaming about being naked in public.

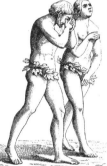

**Needle** A needle can be a symbol of pain but also of repair, so perhaps you are going through a painful situation at the moment but one that is not beyond repair.

**New Year** To dream of the New Year foretells prosperity and happiness in personal relationships. If thinking of the New Year makes you feel tired in your dream, take care not to hook up with the wrong kind of partner in the coming year.

**Nun** A nun in a dream means you will have peace of mind in the near future.

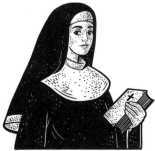

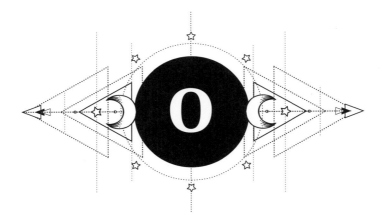

**Obituary** Reading your own obituary in a dream doesn't mean you are going to die, but it is likely to mean that you are underestimating yourself or that you have low self-esteem. Being forced to read about your accomplishments and about how people loved you makes you realize how important you are to others.

**Office** Dreaming about your work office is to admit that you are doing too much. You are overworked and finding it difficult to separate work from home. It's time to take some leave!

**Old Lady** Dreaming of an old lady indicates a need for a touch of wisdom and common sense in your conscious life.

**Old Man** An old man in a dream is symbolic of happiness for the family.

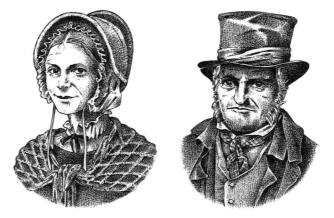

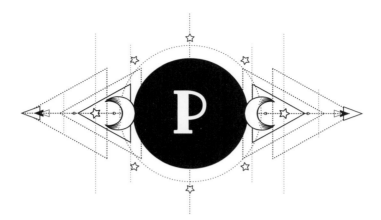

**Packing**  Big changes in your life are predicted if you dream about packing cases or boxes. You might be packing away old problems and worries or boxing up good memories to take with you, but you are certainly leaving an old scene for new beginnings.

**Pain**  Sometimes our dreams can warn us about health problems, and this is particularly true of dreams about specific pain. You should consider having a doctor check you out if you regularly dream about pain in the same part of your body.

**Palm Tree**  Seeing a palm tree in your dream is a hopeful sign as it suggests a time of happiness is on the way to you. Walking down an avenue of palms foretells a cheerful and comfortable home and a faithful partner, but if the palms are dying, there will be sad news.

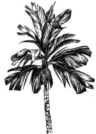

**Paper**  Clean paper indicates that your status is improving, but dirty paper shows that you will suffer injustice.

**Parachute**  There are several ways to look at a dream about parachutes. On one hand, a parachute can be seen to be protective, embracing you with a security blanket; on the other hand, it could symbolize that it is time for you to get yourself out of a situation or to give up an old habit. If you are having difficulty getting a parachute open as you fall down to earth, it suggests that you are being let down by someone you trust.

**Parcel** If you dream of a parcel being delivered to you, someone you haven't seen for a while will pay you a visit. People may also give you back the money that they owe you. If you carry a parcel, you will soon have a difficult job to do, and to let a parcel fall means that a business deal won't go through.

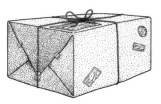

**Parrot** A parrot is often a symbol of gossip or careless talk—maybe you are guilty of this yourself? It could mean that you are the subject of gossip and you need to beware.

**Peacock** A beautiful peacock indicates that wealth is coming to you from the family.

**Police Officer** A police officer appearing in your dream doesn't mean that someone is about to arrest you; it is more likely to indicate that you are about to experience a period of peace and safety after a hectic or difficult time.

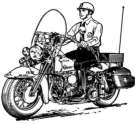

**Postal Carrier** Long-awaited news is about to be delivered if a letter carrier appears in your dream.

**Poverty** Paradoxically, a dream about living in poverty is likely to indicate that there will be a change for the better soon.

**Presents** A dream in which you receive lots of presents means that you are about to experience a setback. Caution will be needed, but it can also be a warning not to get into a situation that will be difficult to live with.

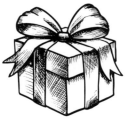

**Purse** If the purse is full, there will be a slight loss, but if it is empty, there will be an unexpected gain.

# PREGNANCY AND DREAMS

Pregnant women often report having multiple vivid dreams. It is not just that the number of dreams increases during pregnancy, but the ability to remember these dreams also improves. This increase might be due to an expectant mother sleeping or napping more due to tiredness, or it might be a result of hormonal changes.

Typical dreams experienced by pregnant women are as follows:

- **Anxiety dreams.** An expectant mother often has extra worries, anxieties, and stresses. She may worry about being a first-time parent, juggling motherhood with work, or concerns over finances. Whatever the root of the anxiety, it is likely to lead to dreams that mirror the feelings that the expectant mother has in her conscious life.

- **Pregnancy or motherhood-related dreams.** The fact that a pregnant woman is probably thinking about her pregnancy or childbirth or her forthcoming baby during her waking hours heightens the probability of her having dreams about motherhood and pregnancy. These dreams might be about the woman's baby talking to her, or about knowing the gender of the baby, or even about the baby being grown up.

- **Nightmares.** Pregnancy nightmares are not uncommon. These are typically triggered by hormone changes and increased emotions while pregnant and can be connected to fear of giving birth or of something going wrong during the birth. Women have also reported dreaming of dropping their babies, of drowning them, or of accidentally choking them. Others have reported nightmares about being lost, trapped, or buried alive.

First-time mothers or those who have experienced traumatic pregnancies or miscarriages in the past are most likely to experience regular, uncomfortable dreams that leave feelings of dread, fear, and anxiety on waking. A change in dreams while pregnant is completely normal and should not cause concern. Bad dreams can sometimes be avoided by following the usual stress-relieving steps before bedtime, such as a warm bath, a social media blackout in the hour before bedtime, a reduction in caffeine and spicy food, for example—and perhaps avoid eating cheese before going to bed.

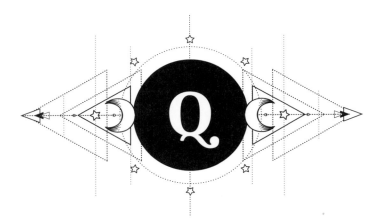

**Quarantine** You may be put into a difficult position by those who do not have your best interests at heart. It might also be a warning of actual quarantine, due to being unwell.

**Quest** A quest represents the stages that you have to go through to achieve your goals in your conscious world. Obstacles and hurdles exist, but you must get around them somehow, and while things will be difficult, the results will be worth it.

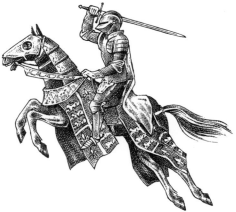

**Quicksand** Dreaming that you are drowning in quicksand indicates that you are feeling overwhelmed at the moment—perhaps with work or with emotions. You are letting things get on top of you, and you need to ask for help.

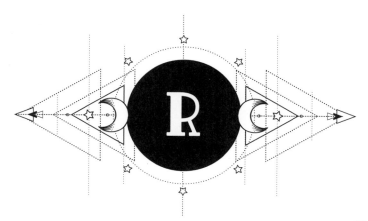

**Rabbit** Luck, abundance, success, magic, and maybe a little bit of romantic love are all things that might be coming your way if a rabbit features in your dream. If the rabbit is white, then you can be reassured about the love of your partner, but a black rabbit points to a fear of intimacy. If the rabbit is hopping, then you can expect some baby news in the near future.

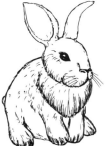

**Race** Dreaming that you are in a race highlights your competitive spirit. Perhaps you are involved in something at work at the moment that has you in competition with a colleague or with another company. On the other hand, dreaming about racing can indicate that you are doing too much at the moment or that you are worried about running out of time with a particular project.

**Rain** Rain symbolizes forgiveness and a new start, literally as if it were washing bad things away. To hear rain or to watch rain has a spiritual connotation, perhaps indicating that you are becoming more aware of your spiritual side.

**Railway Station** A railway station typically indicates that there is a journey to come.

**Rainbow** A brighter future is predicted if you dream about a rainbow, and to dream of a double rainbow is indicative of a financial windfall in the near future. It can also predict unusual events to come and suggest that things are looking up generally. In matters of love, this is a good omen for happiness and success. Good fortune, hope, money, success, happiness—what's not to like about having a rainbow appear in a dream? A rainbow can also symbolize a bridge from your conscious being to your spiritual being, indicating a growing recognition of your spiritual awareness.

**Rats** A rat in your dream is a sign of feelings of guilt, sadness, or envy, suggesting that you take some time to identify your true feelings about a present situation. It may be a warning not to trust a "rat" who comes into your life.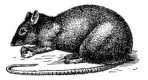

**Reflection** Have you had a dream where you see your own reflection? This indicates that it is time to look at yourself honestly, including the good and the bad. It isn't a reason to beat yourself up over your flaws but an opportunity to learn from them and work out how to make them better. It is also a chance for you to appreciate the good things about your character and personality. Have you dreamed of not being able to see your reflection in a mirror? That would indicate that you have recently lost some of your self-identity or that you are changing yourself and maybe even losing some part of yourself for the benefit of someone else. To see someone else's reflection instead of your own points to you not knowing who you are at the moment—indicating, again, a need for some self-reflection.

**Rose** Social success is on the way, and you should move up the social ladder.

**Running Late** Dreaming about running late for something is an extremely common dream, and it can have several different interpretations. It can mean, for example, that you are currently struggling to live up to the expectations of other people or of yourself. It can also mean that you are worried about missing out on something or even worried about getting older. Finally, it can also be seen as a kind of wake-up call, and a sort of "pull yourself together before it is too late" warning.

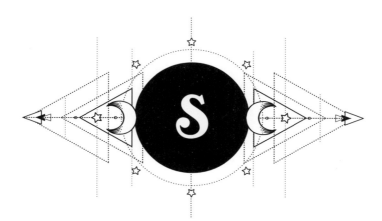

**Sad** A dream in which you are sad may be a reflection of how you are feeling in the conscious world. It is an indication that you need to identify those things that make you happy and focus more on them, while attempting to remove those things from your life that are making you sad.

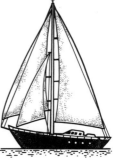

**Sailing** A dream about sailing tends to show how life is currently going for you. If the boat is sailing on smooth seas, then your life at the moment is likely to be "smooth sailing." If, on the other hand, the boat is sailing through stormy weather and treacherous seas, then the same might be an accurate description of your conscious life.

**Sailor** Difficulty or delays in plans are predicted if you dream about a sailor. This can also predict a long and exciting journey, but it can also warn of separation from a lover, possibly due to upsetting the lover by flirting with others too much.

**Salt** In many traditions, salt is seen as protection from evil, so dreams of salt might indicate a need to take care and to seek protection.

**Sapphire** Dreaming of a sapphire indicates a gain or a windfall, and also a good choice of lover.

**School** A feeling of inadequacy or bad experiences at school might lead to a dream that features a school. If, in your dream, you are sitting in a classroom during a lesson, you may well be learning something new in your conscious life or even experiencing a spiritual awakening. Running away from a school is a metaphor for trying to run away from something or someone in your conscious life. If in your dream your school is in ruins—perhaps burnt to the ground or demolished—you are likely to have some unresolved issues or worries from childhood that need to be confronted.

**Scorpion** Dreamed of being stung by a scorpion? Is there currently a situation in your life where bitter words are being uttered? Are negative thoughts and deeds being aimed at you in your conscious life? Or maybe you are currently on a self-destructive path and need to pull yourself back. Scorpions are also symbolic of death and rebirth—perhaps it is time to welcome something new into your life.

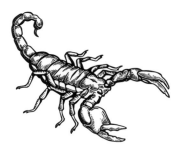

**Scream** Pent-up anger, fear, frustration, and difficulty in communicating with someone are all potential reasons for dreaming about you screaming.

**Seagulls** On one hand, dreaming about seagulls can be a metaphor for strength and powerfulness, but on the other hand, a seagull can also symbolize a need to get away from things, from your everyday life and problems, and such a dream might denote that you need a break.

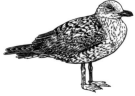

**Searching** If your dream involved you in search of something, the indication is that there is something missing from your life. It might be love, friendship, a sense of peace, or knowledge.

**Seashells** Seashells symbolize protection and hidden things. Perhaps you are hiding something from someone as a form of self-protection, or perhaps you are being advised to keep your own counsel.

**Sex**  To dream about sex does not necessarily indicate the obvious! It may just be a physical reaction to relaxing that sets off the sexual feelings. Apparently, this is more likely to happen if you sleep on your front due to the pressures on the sexual organs. However, other possibilities are that you need to feel close to someone or to feel attractive to someone. If you dream about having sex with someone you know (but who isn't a romantic partner of yours), it does not mean that you want to have sex with them (even though you might feel a little embarrassed the next time you see them) but is more likely to mean that you want the opportunity to get to know them (platonically) better.

**Shampoo**  If you are shampooing your own hair, this is a warning that you are in danger of doing too much to please others and that you are forgetting that you also have needs of your own. If someone else is giving you a shampoo, you will soon make a secret journey that will bring you joy, but you will have to keep the outcome of this from your family and friends.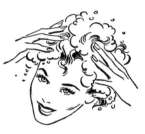

**Shooting Star**  Success in every way is indicated if you dream of a shooting star.

**Sky**  The night sky means temporary difficulties, while a starry sky foretells great changes to your way of life.

**Sleeping Child**  A dream about a sleeping child indicates that good luck is coming.

**Snow**  Generally speaking, dreaming of snow is not great, as there are a variety of relatively unpleasant possibilities, such as looking ill even if you don't actually feel sick, being disappointed in life, and even unable to enjoy something that should be pleasant. Dirty snow is not good for your reputation, while skiing or sledding means choosing the wrong kind of lover. However, melting snow turns unhappiness into joy, which shows that not everything is bad where snow dreams are concerned.

# SNAKE DREAMS

Like them or loathe them in real life, dreaming about a snake or group of snakes is not necessarily comfortable or pleasant. Snakes can be seen as symbols of both healing and hidden danger, so before you relax or freak out about your own snake dream, it might be a good idea to look more into the symbolism of snakes.

Are there snakes everywhere in your dream? This is said to be symbolic of unconscious fears that may have been increasing lately. Does the snake have two heads? This shows there is a conflict in your life at the moment and disagreement that needs to be sorted out. Is your dream about being bitten by a snake? This is a common dream and is something of a bad omen because it is warning you to protect yourself from people, situations, or things that pose an immediate danger to you. The question is where you have been bitten in your dream.

Check out the following possibilities:

- **From behind** This warns of an attack that will catch you off guard or be carried out by people whose identity you are unaware of.
- **The hand** This is connected to deceitful friends, and people whom you trust but who are going to betray you. If the bite is on the right hand, then you can expect this betrayal to come from someone you are close to, but a bite on the left hand means someone who isn't so close to you, but whom you still had trust in.
- **The face** This predicts a personal attack. If the bite is close to your mouth or your throat, it could mean that someone wants to keep you quiet, so perhaps you have been talking too much for their liking.
- **The foot** A snake bite on the foot is symbolic of your movements being restricted. You might find obstacles in your path or that your ambitions are being blocked by someone.
- **A snake in your hair** This is indicative that you might be getting caught up in your thoughts too much. It is a sign to pay more attention to who and what is around you.

There is also much that can be interpreted by the location of the snake in your dream:

- **In bed** This often has sexual connotations. It may be saying that you need to explore your repressed sexuality and desires more.
- **Under the bed** This relates to things that are hidden or dangers that you are unaware of.
- **In the house** This shows that some kind of trouble is very close to home.

What is the snake doing in your dream?

- **Chasing you** If a snake is chasing you, it is likely that you are running away from something. You might also be trying to avoid something in your life, or something about yourself that you'd rather not acknowledge.
- **Swimming in water** This represents a threat to your emotional stability.
- **Snake in a car** This is symbolic of your path ahead—there is the possibility that something or someone will try to get in your way.
- **Killing the snake** If you dream you are killing a snake, then you are able to assert yourself against the threat and you can beat it.
- **Shedding skin** If you dream that a snake is shedding its skin, it is a possible omen of death and rebirth. The process, called ecdysis, can be translated to mean new growth, change, and transformation occurring in your mind, such as shedding the negative aspects so that the new and positive can develop.
- **Snake eggs** Sometimes snake eggs appear in dreams when change is about to occur.
- **Snake turning into a human** A snake that turns into a human can suggest a transformation or a possible underlying threat.
- **Wrapped around your body** This is a symbol of healing or rebirth. If the snake is posing a threat, it can suggest the people who drain you.
- **A snake that is eating or swallowing** These dreams might be a symbol of personal transformation.
- **Crossing your path** When a snake crosses your path or you are aware of its presence, this warns that danger lurks around you. There might be dangerous people close to you whom you might not necessarily deem a threat.

The color of the snake:

- **Red** Anger, emotions, passion, rage, blood, and lust.
- **Green** Envy, greed, finances, harmony, renewal, and growth.
- **Yellow** Intellect, caution, and jealousy.
- **Black** The shadow or dark side of your nature or unknown threats hiding in the shadows.
- **White** Purity, innocence, transformation, light, and safety.
- **Brown** Connects you to the earth, Mother Nature, feminine energy.
- **Orange** Bright, witty, spontaneous, generous, optimistic, eager, and bold.
- **Golden** Connects to the soul or self, a symbol of wisdom and knowledge.
- **Purple** Power, creativity, wisdom, dignity, grandeur, arrogance, and royalty.

**Spending Money**  Take care because there may be extra expenses or losses in the near future.

**Spider**  Quarrels ahead. Someone may be lying in wait for you.

**Strawberries**  Dreaming of strawberries is a good omen for getting on in life and having good times in the future, and suggests you will achieve one heartfelt desire. Eating strawberries means falling in love with someone who isn't interested in you, while growing and selling them means having an abundance of the things you need and want in life.

**Sun**  Success rewards efforts, exams will be passed, goals will be achieved.

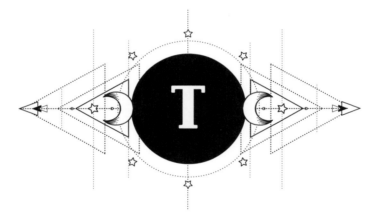

**Tapestry**  A tapestry is symbolic of luxury, comfort, and elegance. To dream of one that is torn and damaged is indicative of a feeling that you want these luxuries but can't afford them at the moment.

**Tarantula**  Your dark, dangerous, sinister side is symbolized by a tarantula. To dream about one may indicate that you have not been your nicest or friendliest to others lately and that you need to show them your nicer side.

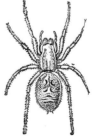

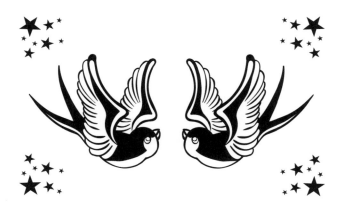

**Tattoo** As with tattoos in real life, this is often symbolic of creativity or a desire to stand out from the crowd—perhaps you are feeling restrained in your conscious life at the moment and unable to express yourself. The nature of the tattoo can also be relevant. A dragon tattoo indicates that you want to be noticed, while the ace of diamonds indicates that you are proud of your recent achievements and want others to acknowledge them.

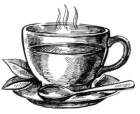

**Tea** Peace, tranquility, serenity, rest, and relaxation are all terms that come to mind when dreaming about drinking a cup of tea. It might be an acknowledgment that you have been really busy lately with hardly any time to stop or pause. If the dream involves you observing a tea ceremony or visiting a tea plantation, then you are feeling adventurous and are ready for an adventure. Reading tea leaves in the dream is a recognition of your developing spiritual awareness.

**Tea Bag** Perhaps less sophisticated than actual tea, a dream in which tea bags appear is an encouragement for you to take some time to relax and recuperate after a period of high stress.

**Teacher** To dream about a teacher of yours—past or future—indicates you currently need advice or assistance about something. It could also mean you are seeking acceptance for something.

**Teeth**  Dreaming about losing all your teeth is another very common theme, and this has multiple potential meanings. It might mean that you are afraid of losing your attractiveness or that you are worried about your appearance. On a deeper level, having a dream where you lose all your teeth may reveal a concern about your communication skills, or there may have been a recent incident when you spoke out and said something you shouldn't have.

**Telegram**  Unexpected news can be expected if a telegram appears in your dream. The news should be good.

**Tiger**  Hidden danger threatens you when a tiger appears in your dream.

**Tomb**  Dreaming about a tomb might make you think of negative things, but it actually indicates a long and happy life is ahead of you.

**Travel**  An impending journey of importance is indicated if you dream of some form of travel.

**Trees**  Dreaming about trees can have a couple of interpretations. On one hand it can indicate that an ambition will be realized, but if the tree has been cut down, a parting from a loved one is likely. A dream about trees can also indicate that some spiritual or intellectual growth is likely to take place in your life in the near future.

**Tunnel**  If someone close to the dreamer is unwell, they will need all the help they can get to pull through: that is the unfortunate message conveyed by a dream in which a tunnel is a feature.

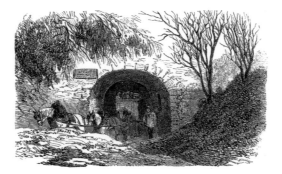

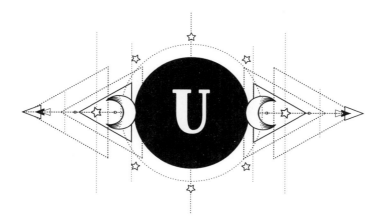

**UFO** A UFO in a dream symbolizes a desire for spiritual awareness. Perhaps you are beginning to develop an interest in spirituality. Another alternative is that you are feeling excluded or alienated from others at the moment, as if you are marginalized from family, friends, or work colleagues.

**Ulcer** This relates to a temporary difficulty that will soon be eased.

**Unconscious** To dream that you are unconscious indicates that you are beginning to acknowledge to yourself that you have been operating for a while in the dark about something. Perhaps you have been ignoring the obvious. This type of dream is a sign to open your eyes and be honest with yourself about what is going on.

**Underground** A desire to isolate yourself from others for a while is often the reason for dreaming about being underground. Perhaps you are feeling overwhelmed or crowded by too many people who have an opinion about your life. Perhaps what you need is to step back from your social world for a moment and just listen to yourself rather than to other people.

**Undressing** Lack of foresight will cause problems if you dream that you are undressing, especially if you do so in public in the dream.

**Unemployed** If you dream that you are unemployed, it is an indication that you are currently feeling underappreciated, worthless, or as if you don't have any purpose in life. It is time to start appreciating yourself for the skills and qualities that you do have.

**Urination** Dreaming about urination can have several meanings. On one hand, it can mean that you are successfully releasing the negativity that you hold, but it could show that you aren't in control of your situation. If you dream of urinating in public, you want people to know that your personal life is nothing to do with them. Finally, you might wake up and discover that you actually need to visit the bathroom!

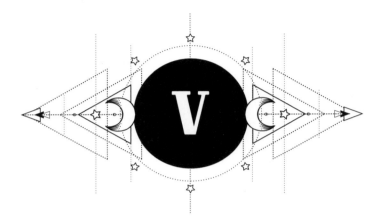

**Venom** Venom in a dream is symbolic of anger, negative emotions, and destructive behavior that is aimed at the dreamer by another person. Perhaps it is time to face the truth about someone you thought you were close to.

**Vermin** Hordes of rats, mice, and other vermin in a dream indicate that you are feeling betrayed by people around you at the moment. You don't know who to trust and are afraid of putting your trust in the wrong person. It can also mean that you are beset by problems, although none of them are really big ones.

**Victim** To be a victim in your dream is actually an empowering position that is designed to make you feel confident about standing up for yourself in real life.

**Violence** To dream about being violent to someone else is a sign that you are harboring pent-up anger toward someone. You have an overwhelming need to express yourself toward that person. If the violence is directed at yourself, it is an indication that you need to be honest with yourself about your relationships with others and withdraw from those that are causing you pain.

**Volcano** Are you boiling over with rage or likely to erupt in anger at something that has been annoying you for a long time? This could be a reason you are dreaming of a volcano, especially one that is erupting. To dream of a dormant volcano shows that you are finally finding a little peace after a vicious argument, or perhaps you have decided that you are not going to be bothered by someone in particular any longer.

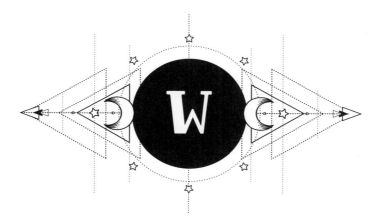

**Waiting** If, in your dream, you are waiting impatiently for something or someone, you are likely to be a controller who likes everything to go the way you had planned. On the other hand, if you are waiting patiently, you are more likely to accept that things happen in their own time and according to their own rhythm, and there is no need to rush.

**Walking** A dream where you are walking can have a myriad of meanings, depending on *how* you are walking. Walking in circles points to your feeling in your conscious life that you are getting nowhere with a problem or an issue. Walking barefoot is symbolic of wanting to feel free or be free of something that has been weighing you down. Walking fast? This is likely to indicate that you have a sudden purpose in life and are eager to get started on something. Walking slowly points to you needing to take time to think things over before you rush into something.

**War** Inner conflict or turmoil or not knowing which side to take in an argument between friends and family are all indicated by dreams of being at war. At the same time, if you dream of being a peacemaker during a war, you probably feel like you are caught between two different sides and are under pressure to pick a side.

**Washing**  Washing signifies cleansing and purifying. To dream that you are washing yourself or your clothes indicates a desire for a new start or to be rid of some trouble that has been bothering you recently. If you are washing your hair, then you are likely to be feeling the need to be rid of negative thoughts and emotions.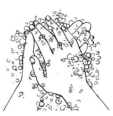

**Water**  Clear water predicts prosperity and good health, but muddy water warns of danger from disputes. Hot water is a warning of danger while cold water is an indication that you need to stop and take stock of a particular situation.

**Waves**  Waves are symbolic of emotional disturbance, with the dreamer oscillating between calmness and panic. A dream about waves suggests a need to take a deep breath, calm down, and decide what direction you want to go.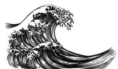

**Weather**  Dreaming about the weather is closely aligned with your current emotional state of mind. Rain represents sadness and depression, while cloudy skies signify a feeling of being downhearted or fed up. Stormy or windy weather denotes conflict and aggression between you and others. Sun, rainbows, and settled weather point to you being happy and content at the moment.

**Well**  Hidden ambitions, abilities, and emotions are represented by dreams that feature a well. The dream indicates a need to bring these things to the surface so that you can start capitalizing on them.

**Wheel**  If a wheel forms part of your dream, then a change for the better is indicated for you in the near future.

**Window**  An open window shows that a problem will soon be solved, while a closed one warns of unexpected danger, but you should be safe. A broken window signifies that a friendship or partnership has been ruined and can't be mended.

**Witch**  Witches are symbolic of sneakiness, bad omens, and trouble brewing. A dream about witches warns of difficulties in the near future. You need to be aware of what others are up to.

# WEDDING DREAMS

It wouldn't be surprising if you were to dream about weddings if you happen to be planning one for yourself, but these can turn up at any time and for any person. Here are some common wedding dreams and their possible meanings:

- **Getting married to a stranger or a friend**—Don't worry, this doesn't mean that you really are going to marry a stranger or a friend! It is more likely to be a sign that either you are going to get closer to a friend who was previously more of an acquaintance, or you are about to make a new friend.
- **Attending a wedding or being invited to a wedding**—This type of dream shows that you are currently feeling the need to meet up with old friends and family members. Perhaps you haven't socialized or caught up with anyone for a while, and you now have an overwhelming need to do so. Go ahead and make that call.
- **Worries about the wedding dress, cake, veil, or ring**—If you are getting married and planning a wedding, then this type of dream is a natural byproduct of having a lot to keep on top of, along with the stress and anxiety about the big day. If you *aren't* getting married but still have this type of dream, it is a reflection of general stress and worry in your life. Whatever the case, it is an indication that you need to stop worrying over the little things and look at the big picture.
- **The groom not showing up**—Again, if you are getting married, to dream that the groom gets cold feet and doesn't turn up is a natural reflection of the stress and anxiety that you are feeling in the run-up to the big day. If you are not getting married, it means that you don't trust someone in your life or you don't know whether you can trust them. Perhaps you have been picking up on subtle clues that they are going to let you down.
- **The wedding meal and reception**—To dream about the wedding meal and reception is indicative of your current attitude toward socializing. If everything goes well at the meal and reception and people are happy and you feel good, then you probably welcome the opportunity to socialize with a lot of people. If, on the other hand, the reception and meal is not a success and is marred by arguments and disagreements and you feel uncomfortable, it is likely a sign that you would rather not socialize at the moment and need some reflective time on your own.

**Wolf** There are two common interpretations of a dream about wolves. On one hand, such a dream warns of underhanded and disloyal behavior by friends or family. On the other hand, there may be business losses to come.

**Worms** Worms suggest that you are worried and anxious, although the worries might be small. They might also point to a feeling of not being recognized for the skills you have and a general sense of being ignored within the workplace.

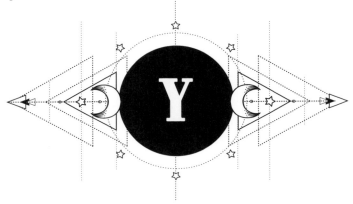

**Yelling** If you are yelling in your dream but no sound is coming out, then you are likely to feel that no one is listening to you at the moment. Perhaps you have a lot to say but no one is asking for your opinion. If there is sound to your yells, you are trying to communicate feelings and emotions that you have kept repressed for a long time.

**Yellow** This bright and sunny color is associated with learning and the intellect. It is also associated with having the kind of personal power that prevents others from walking all over you.

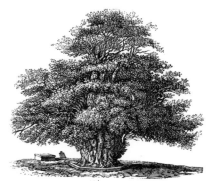

**Yew Tree** Although this tree is associated with graveyards, it has a connection to longevity, because a yew tree can live a long time.

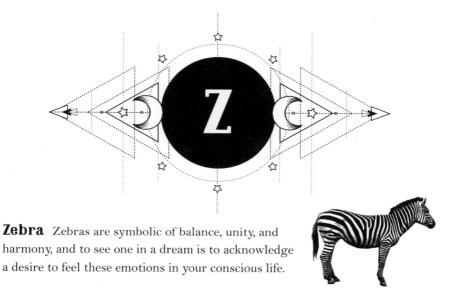

**Zebra** Zebras are symbolic of balance, unity, and harmony, and to see one in a dream is to acknowledge a desire to feel these emotions in your conscious life.

**Zombie** This shows that you feel detached from reality and as though you are simply going through the motions of everyday life. Perhaps you feel a lack of connection to other people or that people are not acknowledging your presence. These are all feelings that are shown by dreaming about being a zombie or being surrounded by zombies.

**Zoo** To dream of visiting a zoo shows mixed fortunes. Some enemies will try to do you harm while others won't be able to do much damage to you. You will travel soon and learn a lot by doing so.

❋ ❋ ❋

# 7

# DREAMS
# IN LITERATURE
# AND ART

rtists and writers know that inspiration can be hard to find, but sometimes the mind will work on the problem while you are asleep, and then a remembered dream brings the answer. And sometimes a dream is itself the answer, such as when Lewis Carroll makes his fantastical world seem plausible because it all happens in the dreaming mind of the young girl Alice.

Here are some famous examples of dreams appearing in Western works of fiction and art.

## In Literature

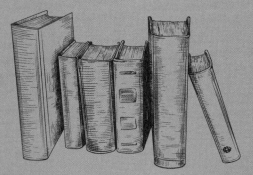

"To die, to sleep—to sleep, perchance to dream—ay, there's the rub, for in this sleep of death what dreams may come ..."
—William Shakespeare (*Hamlet*).

Dreams are a common feature in both modern and classical literature. They can serve as a useful narrative device to authors in that they can disclose information about a character. Through a dream, readers are able to find out the innermost thoughts of the main protagonist, including their wants, desires, and fears. Dreams are also useful for foreshadowing things that might happen during the story or for revealing a flashback that will be of relevance to the plot.

### *1984*, George Orwell

In George Orwell's dystopian novel *1984*, every aspect of Winston Smith's life is under constant surveillance by the state. He, and the rest of the population, cannot speak or associate freely; movement is restricted and always observed, and even talking to yourself will be overheard by the all-seeing and all-hearing telescreen. An aspect of Smith's life that cannot be controlled by the state is his dreams. One example is when he dreamed that he was walking through a pitch-dark room, and someone sitting to one side of him had said as he passed: "We shall meet in the place where there is no darkness."

### *Wuthering Heights,*
### Emily Brontë

Fitting for a gothic novel, the dreams that
we encounter in *Wuthering Heights* are of the
supernatural kind. This is especially true of
Lockwood's dream where Catherine appears as a
ghost who forevermore will haunt the house and
ensure that no one is happy.

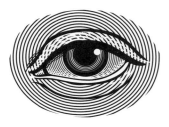

There are also several occasions in the book in which the characters are
guided by their dream; for example, Catherine accepts a marriage proposal after
dreaming about going to heaven:

> I have dreamt in my life, dreams that have stayed with me ever
> after, and changed my ideas; they have gone through and through
> me, like wine through water, and altered the color of my mind.
> And this is one: I'm going to tell it—but take care not to smile at
> any part of it.

### *A Christmas Carol,*
### Charles Dickens

Scrooge is visited by a range of dreamlike apparitions during the story, all
of which teach the old man something about compassion or kindness or
generosity. Happily, these visions have a positive effect on him, and Dickens
gives us a happy ending!

### *A Midsummer Night's Dream,*
### William Shakespeare

Of course, with "dream" in the title, you might
expect that this classic Shakespeare play will feature
a significant amount of dreaming. But as Bottom
indicates, the author may not put much stock in the
meanings of dreams: "I have had a dream, past the wit
of man to say what dream it was. Man is but an ass if
he goes about expounding this dream."

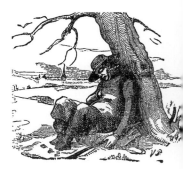

And of course, all is explained when Puck tells us
at the end of the play that the whole performance had
been nothing but a dream.

## *Jane Eyre,*
## Charlotte Bronte

Despite Jane Eyre being so dismissive of fantasies and dreams, the novel is full of references to important dreams and daydreams. For example, there is a scene in which Rochester praises Jane on the quality of her three watercolor landscapes and Jane claims that "the subjects had risen vividly on my mind," to which Rochester replies, "I dare say that you did exist in a kind of artist's dreamland while you blent and arranged these."

## *Oliver Twist,*
## Charles Dickens

Dickens has an interesting commentary to make on what he calls "a drowsy state":

> There is a drowsy state, between sleeping and waking, when you dream more in five minutes with your eyes half-open, and yourself half conscious of everything that is passing around you, than you would in five nights with your eyes fast closed, and your senses wrapped in perfect unconsciousness. At such time, a mortal knows just enough of what his mind is doing, to form some glimmering conception of its mighty powers, its bounding from earth and spurning time and space, when freed from the restraint of its corporeal associate.

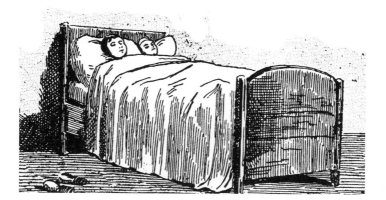

## "Kubla Khan,"
## Samuel Taylor Coleridge

Coleridge used opium to ease an ailment, and the dream he had while in an opium-induced trance led him to write his famous poem "Kubla Khan."

## "The Raven,"
## Edgar Allan Poe

> Deep into that darkness peering, long I stood there wondering, fearing,
> Doubting, dreaming dreams no mortals ever dared to dream before.

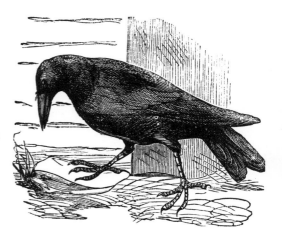

The classic gothic poem by Edgar Allan Poe depicts a man who, on the edge of deep sleep, is interrupted by a tapping of a door but finds nothing or no one on the other side. What follows is a monologue dedicated to an ebony raven who becomes the main character in the poem. Literary critics are divided on whether the raven represents a dream or whether it is a symptom of grief.

## *Rebecca,*
## Daphne du Maurier

> Last night I dreamt I went to Manderley again. It seemed to me I stood by the iron gate to the drive, and for a while I could not enter, for the way was barred to me.

This opening line to the famous novel *Rebecca,* is one of the most foreshadowing openings to any novel. The narrator's entry to Manderley is indeed barred to her, metaphorically at least, by the ghostlike presence of Rebecca. The opening is also an indication of the importance that dreams will play in the story.

## *The Invisible Man,* H. G. Wells

A famous quote from *The Invisible Man* by H. G. Wells is a good example of the fine line that characters can take between being totally immersed in a dream and aware that it is a fiction: "In the middle of the night, she woke up dreaming of huge white heads like turnips, that came trailing after her, at the end of interminable necks, and with vast black eyes. But being a sensible woman, she subdued her terrors and turned over and went to sleep again."

## *Treasure Island,* Robert Louis Stevenson

Robert Louis Stevenson dreamed about *The Strange Case of Dr. Jekyll and Mr. Hyde* and wrote the book shortly afterward. But let's leave the last literary word on dreams to *Treasure Island ...*

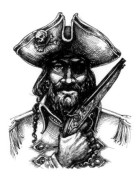

> Many the long night I've dreamed of cheese—toasted, mostly.

# In Art

Since the Middle Ages, artists have sought to create images of dreams, fantasies, and nightmares. Renaissance artists, during the fourteenth to sixteenth centuries, drew inspiration from ancient Greek and Roman philosophers to try to visualize what happens when we sleep. In the seventeenth and eighteenth centuries, the attention of Enlightenment artists moved to reason and rationality and their impact on dreams. In the nineteenth century, the Symbolist and Romanticist movements used eroticism,

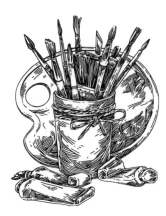

fantasy, and even death to represent dreams. The Surrealist movement of the twentieth century broke from the traditions of rationality to produce dream art that lent full rein to creativity and irrationality.

### *The Vision of Tindal* (1520–1530), **Hieronymus Bosch**

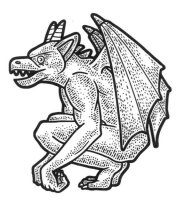

This is a disturbing, almost hallucinatory piece of art inspired by the medieval poem "The Vision of Knight Tindal." The rebellious knight of the poem dreams of a vision of hell and afterward seeks his moral redemption. In the painting, monstrous creatures and a grotesque background depicting hell illustrate the knight's dream or, more accurately, his nightmare.

### *Sleeping Apollo and the Muses with Fame* (1549), **Lorenzo Lotto**

Similarly, this masterpiece depicts a sleeping, naked Apollo. An angel flies overhead while a group of muses perform an inhibited dance.

### *The Sleep of Reason Produces Monsters* (1799), **Francisco de Goya**

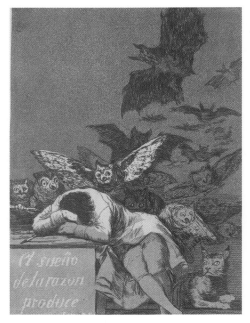

Goya uses images of predatory creatures seen by the Spanish as evil, as a way to criticize what he sees as an irrational, superstitious, and old-fashioned society in need of reform.

### *Nightmare* (1781), **Henry Fuseli**

The painting depicts a woman stretched across her bed with a mythical demon sitting on her chest, and an enormous horse with flaring nostrils poking his head out from behind a curtain. This shocked contemporary audiences and is seen by many as a precursor for Sigmund Freud's psychoanalytical theories.

## *The Sleeping Gypsy* (1897), Henri Rousseau

A woman is sleeping in the desert, and her face is being licked by a passing lion. Things, however, might not be as simple as they seem: is the lion part of the woman's dream or is he real, and therefore, is she in danger? Is she really asleep and dreaming at all, or is the picture itself a dream?

## *Dream Caused by the Flight of a Bee around a Pomegranate a Second before Waking* (1944), Salvador Dalí

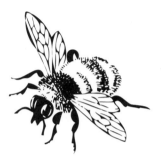

With a title as descriptive as this, you might think it an easy task to guess what this masterpiece depicts. Would you, however, have predicted a naked woman (the artist's wife) sleeping on a rock in the sea, with two tigers and a rifle flying toward her? The tigers and rifle are emerging from the mouth of a fish, itself having emerged from a bursting pomegranate. Oh, and there is also a white elephant on extended legs, carrying what could be a large crystal on his back, walking in the sky above. This is a dream that you would surely remember the next day!

❋ ❋ ❋

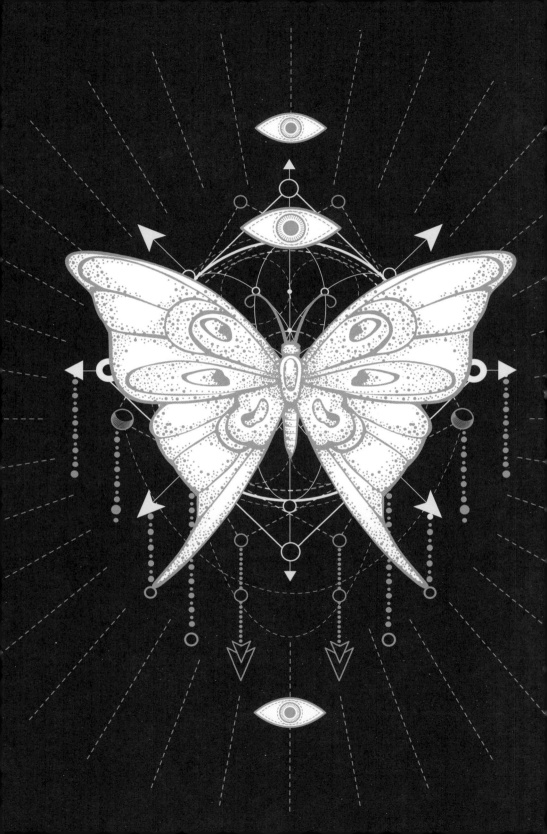

# CONCLUSION

We come to the end of our dream journey, one that has seen us look at the biological, psychological, and mystical reasons we dream. We have learned a little about how the brain works and how it causes us to dream, but we have also been able to find out about how human emotions and experiences influence what we dream about.

From dreams about acorns to nightmares about zombies, we have looked at a plethora of themes, motifs, and symbols that populate our dreams and leave us perplexed in the morning. I hope that this book has helped you be a little less confused about the content of your dreams and has inspired you to try to remember them more often and to act on the messages they are trying to give you.

Good night, sweet dreams!

# INDEX

Note: Terms in **bold** indicate associated dream themes/meanings.

# IMAGE CREDITS